THE
MIRACLE
CARB
DIET

THE MIRACLE CARB DIET

MAKE CALORIES AND FAT DISAPPEAR—WITH FIBER!

Tanya Zuckerbrot, MS, RD

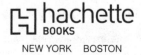

NEW YORK   BOSTON

Copyright © 2012 Tanya Zuckerbrot

Miracle Carb™ is a trademark of F-Factor Group, LLC, and Tanya Zuckerbrot

Cover copyright © 2017 by Hachette Book Group, Inc.

Hachette Books
Hachette Book Group
1290 Avenue of the Americas, New York, NY 10104
hachettebooks.com
twitter.com/hachettebooks

First Edition: December 2012

Hachette Books is a division of Hachette Book Group, Inc. The Hachette Books name and logo are trademarks of Hachette Book Group, Inc.

The publisher is not responsible for websites (or their content) that are not owned by the publisher.

The Hachette Speakers Bureau provides a wide range of authors for speaking events. To find out more, go to www.hachettespeakersbureau.com or call (866) 376-6591.

Library of Congress Cataloging-in-Publication Data

Zuckerbrot, Tanya.
The miracle carb diet: make calories and fat disappear—with fiber!/Tanya Zuckerbrot.
p. cm.
ISBN 978-1-4013-2462-9
1. High-fiber diet.   2. Reducing diets.   3. High-fiber diet—Recipes.
4. Reducing diets—Recipes.   I. Title.
RM237.6.Z85 2012
613.2'63—dc23
2011050557

ISBNs: 978-1-4013-2462-9 (hardcover); 978-1-4013-0433-1 (ebook)

Printed in the United States of America

LSC-C

10 9 8 7 6 5 4

to my Grandma Claire

Contents

THE MIRACLE CARB DIET

INTRODUCTION
THE PROMISE

Chances are you are going to gain weight today.

In this country, if you are not working at losing weight or maintaining your current weight, you are almost guaranteed to gain weight. Why?

We live in an obesogenic society that promotes gaining weight and isn't conducive to weight loss.

Food portions are out of control—what I call portion distortion. Everything from sandwiches and muffins to bags of chips are supersized. Realistically, who trims down their sandwich or counts out a proper portion of crackers? The problem is we've lost sight of what a proper portion looks like. Today, big is the norm; we expect jumbo portions all the time. Advances in food technology are making us fatter, too. Refined foods may look and taste delicious, but modern processing routinely strips away the nutrients that make food filling, especially fiber. Converting potatoes to potato flakes, apples to juice, and wheat to white bread makes it convenient to enjoy them, but the truth is that processed foods don't satisfy hunger for very long.

And this is why we have become a nation of overeaters. In America, if you are hungry, you are in luck, because food is omnipresent. You can grab a bite of almost anything anywhere and any time of the day. Gas stations and drugstores sell food, airports have vast food courts, and many office buildings have a cafeteria or vending machines. It's ironic that the abundance and close proximity of processed food is what keeps us perpetually hungry.

The Centers for Disease Control and Prevention (CDC) estimates that 68 percent of our adult population is either overweight or obese. That's a scary statistic, but you don't have be a part of it. As a registered dietitian who specializes in weight loss, I know you can lose weight and keep it off while eating deliciously and healthfully, without hunger. To prove it, I created the Miracle Carb Diet, which is contrary to any other diet out there. My promise to you is that you can lose weight, all while:

- Eating carbs you love
- Dining out
- Drinking alcohol
- Working out less

Whether you need to lose ten pounds, fifty pounds, or no weight at all, the Miracle Carb Diet is a blueprint for building your best life with an easy, healthy plan for eating the fiber-rich foods that will help you reach and stay at your healthy weight, have more energy, combat the effects of aging, and even live longer. That's right. You'll eat more, weigh less, and live longer!

FIBER: THE MIRACLE CARB

Fifteen years ago, while working as a clinical dietitian, I developed separate diets for diabetic and cardiovascular patients and discovered an unexpected benefit: Everyone improved their medical condition, but they lost weight as well. What was the common denominator between both of the diets? Fiber. It was then that I realized that fiber was nutrition's superhero, improving health and allowing for weight loss without hunger. By now most everyone has pretty much gotten the memo that fiber is good for you, and maybe you're one of those people—and there are many—who assumes you're getting enough by eating a salad for lunch or switching to whole wheat bread. That's a good start, but you're still cheating your body. Just how much fiber you need, how to get it, and how to optimize its benefits remains a mystery for most people. It's my mission to change that. Ignorance isn't going to be an excuse anymore.

To put it simply, fiber is nature's miracle carb.

So much revolutionary research has been done since I wrote *The F-Factor Diet* in 2006, not only validating but greatly advancing those early theories I had about fiber based on the experiences of my own patients. Since then, F-Factor has evolved from being a way to eat to being a way to live, and my new Miracle Carb Diet serves as the action plan for achieving your best self the F-Factor way.

BEST BODY, BEST SELF

I've yet to meet someone who aspires to mediocrity. For me, being a registered dietitian isn't just about making sure the body gets the fuels it needs. It is about nurturing the whole person, because hunger, I've found, is often a symptom of what's missing in our lives. Many turn to food to soothe their souls but end up feeling worse as their weight becomes a problem.

Fair or unfair, we're often judged by our physiques and by the way we project and present ourselves. If you feel unattractive and defeated by your weight, there's a good chance that you are not displaying confidence or sharing the wonderful qualities and true gifts you have to offer a potential employer or mate, friends, family, or your community. The best part of my job is watching the transformation—not just physically but emotionally—in the clients I coach. Seeing people gain confidence and strive to be their best is why I love what I do. I've put that same passion into writing this book.

I want you to think of me as your partner from this moment on. When you try to hike that proverbial Everest by yourself—without the right tools, training, or map—your chances of reaching the summit and achieving success are limited. Through this book, I am here to coach you, support you, cheer you on, and help strategize every step of the way. This book guides you along a path I have carefully charted and know to be the safest, easiest, and surest way to get you to your goals. More than anything, I want you to be able to experience the exhilaration of reaching your goal, of becoming your best possible self, inside and out. If you slip, I will catch you. If you grow weary, I'll show you how to reboot. You will find everything you need to succeed in this book and in yourself. You're already motivated to start this journey, or you wouldn't be here.

All the time that you spend worrying about something related to your weight—agonizing over the problem areas of your body, searching for what you can wear to camouflage them, thinking about what you're going to eat or regret eating—is time I am going to give back to you. Multiply all your negative thoughts and feelings about your weight in a given day by a week, by a month, by every year that you have been unhappy about your body, and then think of how much time that all adds up to. Now envision yourself filling those hours happily playing with your kids, pursuing a hobby, furthering your career, or socializing. Even a single hour spent dwelling on your weight is an hour stolen from a better life. Imagine how liberating it's going to be when you can forever check "lose weight" off your life's to-do list.

WHAT IS THE F-FACTOR WAY?

The F-Factor way is the philosophy and foundation behind the Miracle Carb Diet. It is a way of thinking and living healthfully. Unlike other diets that ask you to starve and cut out food groups like carbs, this nutritionally sound approach to eating for life gives you more choices, not fewer. You won't be asked to ban carbohydrates, proteins, fats, or even alcohol. You will be able to indulge your sweet tooth. And you'll be able to maintain your normal lifestyle. Through the four simple stages of the Miracle Carb Diet, you'll rev up your metabolism, shed pounds, achieve and maintain your target weight, and even defy the aging process. There's nothing extreme about my approach. The key is to combine high-fiber foods with lean protein at every meal. And the amount of fiber we're talking about is simply what the Academy of Nutrition and Dietetics recommends for daily consumption! This diet isn't about tricking your body or shocking the system into a state of semi-starvation. It's actually about routine maintenance: giving your body what it requires to function the way it is supposed to. By definition that's what a diet is: a normal pattern of eating.

A DIFFERENT KIND OF DIET

The beauty of F-Factor's Miracle Carb Diet is that, unlike other diets, you reap the benefits from what you add, not just what you take away. By eating more fiber, you will lose weight. Safely, steadily, naturally. The truth is I can promise better results with "forbidden" foods like bread and chocolate than any fad diet out there. That's because the Miracle Carb Diet isn't about sacrifice or starvation. It's about simplicity and success. And from my vantage point, I know there has never been a better time—or a better battle plan—to lead millions of overweight Americans to victory at last in their struggle to achieve and maintain the healthy bodies they deserve. That *you* deserve. Feeling and looking your best will rock your world—you'll see. By putting your best self out there, your dealings with everyone—your boss and coworkers, friends, mate, children, siblings, even strangers—can't help but be more positive.

Most diets claim to make you thinner, but only the Miracle Carb Diet can claim that you'll lose weight and live longer, too. And we have serious scientific evidence to back this up. A truly groundbreaking study of nearly four hundred thousand people over a ten-year period by the National Institutes of Health (NIH) discovered that those who ate fiber-rich diets lived longest. Fiber was credited with reducing the risk of death from cardiovascular disease, infectious and respiratory disease, and some forms of cancer. Even if you're already at your ideal weight, increasing your fiber intake by following the Miracle Carb Diet will help you maintain your weight, improve your overall health, and increase your chances of living longer as well.

Fiber has rightfully made its way from the fringe to the mainstream; what once was thought of as downright boring or medicinal is now the hottest nutrient around. Moreover, it's a proven solution to a serious problem—epidemic obesity. The good news is that it's easier than ever to follow this family-friendly eating plan, whether you're a passionate foodie who loves to cook, a frequent-flying executive, or a finicky diner who tries to dissect every menu. And guess what? We're not just talking your grandma's prunes anymore; we're talking pasta, soups, sandwiches, even chicken fingers. So raise your glass and toast your success, because on F-Factor, you can drink alcohol right from day one.

This book will serve as a GPS that will lead you to your healthiest, fittest self. F-Factor's Miracle Carb Diet lays forth a clear, comprehensive path for you. From the first bite, you'll learn which foods to eat, when to eat them, and in what combinations to optimize your results, and you can either follow or be inspired by my new collection of more than one hundred recipes, along with my complete shopping lists. This is an eating plan that's filling, flexible, and incredibly food-friendly (that *F* doesn't just stand for fiber, you know).

Most people are savvy enough to realize that excess weight puts them at a higher risk for chronic, often deadly diseases like hypertension and diabetes. Feeling desperate and defeated, they search for a miracle cure, whether it's the latest celebrity cleanse, or potentially dangerous diet pills sold over the Internet, or one of the countless tabloid diets promising to melt away pounds like butter on a hot waffle iron. The problem with fad diets, besides often being flat-out unhealthy, is their failure to keep the weight off once you lose it. Obviously you can't stay on a lemon-water diet for three months, let alone three years. And does wearing a size 8 really mean a slice of bread can never touch your lips again? Do you have to seek closure to your love affair with chocolate? I promise you that is not the case.

I grew up with a Colombian mother, a Jewish father, and a house that was always filled with the delicious aromas of home cooking. My mother's Latin culture meant there was rice on the table at every meal, even if we were having potatoes, too. Fried empanadas and fried plantains were mainstays of my childhood, and my Jewish grandmother handed down her recipes for noodle kugel, fried latkes, and her famous cream cheese pie. But there was always a big bowl of salad on the table, too, and I figured out by my teens that if I filled up on the healthy greens and veggies as a first course, I would be more inclined to show some moderation when it came to the more decadent dishes.

Now, as a mother of three young children, I know how important it is to pass on healthy eating habits to them, so they can grow up without ever having to worry about losing weight. That doesn't mean they have never tasted pizza or are being raised on celery stalks! Trust me, we're doing our part to support the snack industry. I love to cook, and I love to eat, and I would never take away that pleasure from my clients any more than I would from my own family.

In addition to showing you how to incorporate fiber and lean protein into your diet, I'll tell you how to exercise to make the most of the Miracle Carb Diet. If you're trying to get lean and toned by doing cardio exercise on the treadmill, you're running nowhere fast! I have nothing against cardio exercise, because it's a great way to work your heart and clear your head, but weight training is really the perfect complement to a high-fiber diet. It will give you the trim, toned look you've always dreamed of—without having to invest big chunks of time and money in gym memberships, special equipment, or exercise gear. Weight training builds lean muscle mass, which will boost your metabolism far more than cardio ever could.

I'll also describe the biggest diet busters and show you how to maneuver around the dangerous patches of quicksand. You'll learn how to gracefully handle food bullies who try to sabotage you. I'll share the quick tips that have worked for my clients, like how to vanquish an ice cream binge, what hors d'oeuvres to choose at a cocktail party, and what to grab to go at the airport. You'll master the art of piling a bountiful plate at the salad bar and discover how to diminish cravings or ravenous hunger with a strategic carbs-and-protein snack to stabilize your blood sugars.

The Miracle Carb Diet also zeros in on specific food cravings—salty, crunchy, sugary, fatty—and explains both the physiological and psychological reasons behind each, as well as the best defense against them. I will introduce you to many new and improved products to put on your shopping list, such as a delicious variety of yogurts, cheeses, crackers, and even chocolate.

With this book, you will have the resources to eat F-Factor-friendly anytime, anywhere. I'll teach you how to journal, logging what you eat in a way that lets you easily keep track of your progress. Journaling even a few minutes each day makes you accountable for what you put in your mouth, and it will also help you explore emotional eating and discover patterns that may have been sabotaging your best efforts to lose weight. Along the way, you may also unlock hidden strengths you didn't even realize you already have.

I'll also help you maintain control so you won't rely on food for comfort during stressful or anxious times, and show you how you can enjoy the holidays and other celebrations without feeling deprived or left out. You can even build menus for the entire family out of the foods you'll be eating on this plan, without having to prepare a separate diet meal just for yourself. You'll become a master at navigating the Sunday brunch buffet or sushi bar without going off the rails. In fact, armed with some practical new tips, you'll be able to dine out from day one on this plan, and what you learn will become so second nature that even the hardest choices, such as what snacks to grab at a gas station when you're on the go, will be simple.

Getting you through the tough spots is one of my specialties. I'm fascinated by the behavioral component of weight loss and have created a program that recognizes the different combinations of patterns and pitfalls every dieter faces. My work as a dietitian in private practice has given me a unique insight into the psychology of losing weight, whether I'm coaching a celebrity stressing about his public image or a stay-at-home mom yearning to reclaim her identity. Over the years, I've learned how to help motivate people who are struggling with their weight. In this book, I'll channel all that I know to help you succeed. You'll be able to draw from the personal experiences of F-Factor devotees like Jeff, a forty-six-year-old businessman who never cooks for himself and lost more than 50 pounds after his worried wife staged a diet intervention. Or Laura, a lifelong yo-yo dieter who would start out supermotivated, enjoy some dramatic results, then lose steam and sabotage herself with comfort foods until we got her back on track and gave her the quick-recovery toolkit she can use to correct course whenever necessary.

PREPARE TO SUCCEED

Turn on the TV these days and you'll come across any number of popular reality shows focusing on desperate people fighting to lose pounds while a tough-love coach or personal trainer bullies them until they sometimes literally collapse. No wonder the follow-up stories months or years later so often show that whatever weight was lost has been regained and then some. (Who wouldn't get depressed and self-medicate with a hefty dose of cookies 'n' cream after an ordeal like that?)

My philosophy is to approach this boomerang problem with compassion as well as commitment. I will show you how to push past the emotional walls standing in the way of your happiness and well-being. When a client walks through my door, I know that he or she has decided to make a change, just as you have by picking up this book. You are ready to shed unwanted pounds, but you also want to be healthier, live longer, have more energy, and feel sexy and happy. In short, you want to enjoy life to the fullest and not let your weight hold you back. You've already done the toughest prep work by letting yourself be excited by the possibility of real, lasting change.

People who surrender themselves to being overweight use fat to cushion the blow of disappointment they always anticipate; they were just *meant* to be heavy, or their metabolisms won't *let* them take off the pounds they loathe. Going on and off fad diets that don't work in the long term is as harmful to your mind-set as it is to your body: You condition yourself to fail and to accept failure as something you somehow deserve. The F-Factor way is to attack that resistance at its root and empowers you to be your very best self, no matter what your profession, passion, or purpose.

We live in a world where so much is out of our control: the weather is unpredictable; you arrive at the airport and your flight is canceled; your flight is on time, but your luggage does not arrive when you do (yep, I recently spent the first few days of a beach vacation dressed in a Ritz-Carlton robe); sometimes the lady who sells you postage stamps is downright surly. We figure it's all in the hands of whatever higher power we believe in, or, as the popular saying goes, "it just is what it is." It's easy to write off body size in the same way. Easy and 100 percent wrong, because one of the few things in life we do have control over is what we put in our mouths.

Let's get real, people. We all know that was you pulling out of the drive-thru with the bagful of burgers and fries, and it wasn't invisible Girl Scouts who filled your pantry with cookies when Thin Mint season rolled around. Furthermore, no one coerced you into getting the fettuccine in a rich cream sauce instead of grilled wild salmon at the restaurant last night, and that was clearly your voice grandiosely ordering dessert for the entire table. You eat it, you own it.

When it comes to what we eat, the fork is in our hands and ours alone. I don't say this to burden you. I'm saying this to empower you. If you want this badly enough, it's yours for the taking.

The Miracle Carb Diet will inspire you to discover new foods and adopt new habits that will become part of your new and improved lifestyle. You will not only see the results, you will feel them. Your entire relationship with food will change, clearing the path for you to pour your thoughts and energy into all those things you would rather do than obsess about your weight.

You may recall that I began this book by stating that awareness is vital to this process. The reason I say that is because you have to be able to picture your success, and embrace it wholly, in order to achieve it. Success is the outcome of thinking, visualizing, planning, and taking action.

The most brilliant coaches in the world will tell you that their top athletes are all masters of visualization. They don't just see themselves hoisting the winning trophy into the air: They create a mental movie of themselves at peak performance, overcoming their worst physical obstacles or fiercest opponents. When they train, they visualize themselves getting stronger. You can apply that same winning technique to losing weight.

Good things are coming! I have worked with hundreds of patients to lose thousands of pounds. Now my job is to give you the same tools and inspiration. Your success is my success. I believe in the proof I have seen for myself. Nothing works better than fiber and the F-Factor way to achieve a leaner, stronger body. You'll shed unwanted pounds, but that's not all. The weight you lose is going to stay off because you'll have permanent solutions for permanent results.

So that's our basic road map. You are ready to embark on a life-changing journey that will transform you from the inside out. My promise to you is that you will achieve this while eating the carbs you love, dining out and drinking alcohol from day one, and devoting a lot less time to working out.

How great is that? Let's get going!

1

THE MIRACLE CARB: FIBER

"I don't get it. How am I supposed to lose weight on this diet? I'm already eating way less than this, and I'm not losing much at all, so how on earth is adding food going to work?"

Like most new clients, Stacey was a veteran dieter who had watched the numbers on her scale go up and down, then up, up, up again for much of her adult life. At age thirty-eight, the working mother of three was still at odds with the 30 pounds she had gained during her last pregnancy—and the pounds were winning. "My daughter just started first grade!" she said with a sigh. "I've spent the past three months practically starving myself, and I'm still only down six pounds!" I could see the toll Stacey's diet was taking on her: A natural beauty with green eyes and delicate features, Stacey looked tired and defeated. Her skin was sallow, and her red hair was dull and lank. She was in a bad place, and my heart went out to her. She looked at me dubiously as I ticked off all the foods she could be enjoying and tried to explain how by eating more she could wind up weighing less. "How is that even possible?" Stacey wondered. Believe me, that's a question I hear a lot! And it's one that I never tire of answering. Once you have a better idea of how the body digests, utilizes, and stores food, you'll see why some foods are more likely than others to cause weight gain. It's easy to tell you not to eat cake, but you're more likely to pass up a slice if you understand why.

MIRACLE? OR SCIENCE?

You only lose weight if you burn more calories than you consume. Metabolism is the rate at which your body burns calories for energy. If you try to shed pounds by drastically limiting your food intake, or by following a low-calorie diet but eating too many refined foods, you could force your body into starvation mode, and your metabolism will actually slow down as a survival mechanism. Your body can also shift into starvation mode and start storing additional fat if you increase your physical activity to an unhealthy extreme. But the right combination of diet and exercise will leave you lean, fit, and healthier than ever. You'll see how adding fiber to your diet makes a huge difference.

There are a few basic facts that make fiber a weight-loss miracle. Fiber adds bulk to food without adding calories, which make high-fiber foods great for dieting. It also swells in the stomach, slows digestion, and boosts metabolism, and all of this combines to make losing weight the F-Factor way healthier and easier. What really gives fiber its miracle status is the way it soaks up and removes fat and calories in the stomach before your body can absorb them. Incredibly, the fiber found in delicious, nutritious, filling carbs does what no other food can—it actually makes fat and calories disappear!

Fiber-rich foods typically require more chewing, which decreases food intake in a few ways. First, chewing promotes the secretion of saliva in the mouth and gastric juice in the stomach, which results in increased satiety. More chewing takes time, which allows the brain and stomach to communicate that you're getting full. Then there's the benefit from expending energy—you work harder and burn more calories eating an apple than you do eating applesauce or drinking apple juice. Fiber actually boosts your metabolism. So there you have it: Fiber speeds up weight loss, pure and simple.

But this diet is about more than just adding fiber. You must eat protein, vegetables, fruits, and complex carbohydrates, too. From the first day on the Miracle Carb Diet, you can choose from foods like chicken, eggs, turkey, veal, lamb, fish, shrimp, scallops, lobster, and even steak. Clinical evidence has shown fiber and protein in combination work best to keep you feeling full for the longest period of time and on the fewest calories. By concentrating on what you should be adding to your diet instead of what you should be eliminating, you are setting yourself up for success. You go into this knowing you won't ever have to feel hungry or count the minutes—or hours—until you're allowed to eat again.

Granted, this may sound pretty technical, but know that this diet has withstood the most rigorous road test and it's a proven winner.

"Say you're in the market for a new car," I explained to my client Stacey. "You can walk into a car dealership and choose to spend all your money on a sexy sports car with Italian leather seats and a killer sound system. Sure, you'll get plenty of attention showing off that car at first, but then little things start to go wrong, followed by major things. It's exasperating, because you spent all that money for a car and you can't count on it. You end up on the side of road, feeling duped.

"Then there's the Volvo. The Volvo isn't going to make any jaws drop when you pull into the parking lot at work. Volvos have been around for a long time, and they never change much, because, frankly, they don't need to. Volvos do their job, and they do it brilliantly. They're the quiet superachievers. That's what you're getting with the Miracle Carb Diet: a very smart choice."

I can guarantee you right now that fiber is going to be around, doing a brilliant job, long after the flashier diets have crashed and burned. Here's how it works:

There are two types of fiber—soluble and insoluble—and each performs a useful task in our digestive process. Insoluble fiber, commonly known as roughage, is Mother Nature's custodial service, sweeping the digestive tract so everything that has to pass through can keep moving along more quickly. That, in turn, helps reduce your risk of developing diseases like colon cancer and diverticulitis. What makes it a winner for dieters is that eating foods rich in insoluble fiber kicks metabolism into high gear. This type of fiber does not dissolve in water, so the body has to work extra hard to move it through the system and, to do that, the body burns up calories. Common sources for insoluble fiber are dark, leafy greens and cruciferous veggies, such as broccoli, as well as certain fruits, such as apples. Wheat bran and whole grain cereals are also good sources.

Soluble fiber, on the other hand, does dissolve in water. Foods like oats, beans, peas, pears, and oranges all contain soluble fiber. Once inside your stomach, soluble fiber swells up like a sponge and gives a jellylike bulk to food, making you feel full. Soluble fiber also has cholesterol-lowering properties because it binds with cholesterol and pulls it out of the body; it does the same with toxins and estrogen as well, which is why foods rich in soluble fiber are helpful in preventing diseases such as breast cancer.

The rewards at hand aren't limited to better health and increased longevity. Fiber's remarkable cleansing properties have been shown to boost energy and enhance beauty, too—think brighter, clearer complexion, glossier hair, and stronger nails.

It's important to get enough of both soluble and insoluble fiber in your diet on a daily basis. The sad truth is the average American doesn't even come close; the Academy of Nutrition and Dietetics recommends adult women get 25 grams of fiber in their diet each day, and men, 38 grams, yet most of us get only 9 to 11 grams of fiber per day—less than half the recommended amount.

What's great is that it's getting easier to meet our daily fiber needs. Lately, you may have noticed more foods at the supermarket—from cereal, yogurt, and crackers to beverages and even chewing gum—that make "added fiber" claims. The market for foods touting dietary fiber is booming, hitting an estimated $470 million in sales last year. That means you can get more fiber nutrition in your diet by eating familiar and delicious everyday foods, as well as by trying some exciting new ones.

Fiber's rise as a nutritional superstar began in the 1970s when an East African surgeon, Denis Burkitt, sought to explain why common Western ailments such as heart disease, irritable bowel syndrome, and varicose veins were rare in Africa and other third world countries. Through his research, he found that these diseases were least prevalent in cultures where the typical diet was high in fiber and low in refined carbohydrates. Dr. Burkitt also observed that the emergence of those Western diseases coincided with the invention of a new milling technique in the late nineteenth century that removed fiber from whole grain flour to create white flour. Modern food processing, for all its efficiency and quality control, routinely strips nutrients—especially fiber—from the foods that line supermarket shelves.

Over the past few decades, more and more research has validated fiber's importance in the diet for promoting health and preventing obesity and disease. It's truly exciting to me as a dietitian who has made high-fiber nutrition the cornerstone of my practice. Years of experience have shown me how adding fiber back into a person's diet can greatly improve his or her health and quality of life.

The good news about fiber keeps getting better: New research proves that eating more fiber does indeed *speed up* metabolism. A Pomona College study by Sadie Barr and Jonathan Wright determined whole foods rich in dietary fiber require significantly more energy to digest than processed foods that are low in fiber. In layman's terms, that means your body burns more calories digesting a slice of whole grain bread than it does digesting a slice of white bread. Barr fed her test subjects sandwiches made from multi-grain bread with Cheddar cheese and sandwiches made from white bread with processed cheese. Each sandwich contained the same number of calories and comparable amounts of protein, carbohydrates, and fat. When the participants' metabolic rates were measured over a six-hour period, Barr found that it took 50 percent less energy to digest the processed sandwich.

HOW HEALTHY IS "HEALTHY"?

I want you to do a little thought experiment now, and the results will probably surprise you. When I see new clients, I have them write down what they eat on a typical day. Generally, they fall into one of three categories:

PERSON ONE: TYPICAL AMERICAN DIET

BREAKFAST
- Plain bagel with 3 tablespoons of cream cheese
- 1 cup of orange juice

LUNCH

- Overstuffed tuna sandwich on a roll
- 1 bag of potato chips
- 1 can of Diet Snapple

SNACK

- 2 chocolate chip cookies
- 1 cup of coffee with half-and-half creamer

DINNER

- 1 cup of wonton soup
- 1 cup of beef and broccoli
- 1 cup of white rice
- 1 fortune cookie
- Diet Coke

DESSERT

- 1 scoop of vanilla ice cream

PERSON TWO: HIGH-FIBER DIET

BREAKFAST

- Whole-wheat English muffin with 1% cottage cheese
- 6-ounce container fat-free plain Greek yogurt
- 1 cup of raspberries
- Coffee with splash of skim milk

LUNCH

- Large salad with non-starchy vegetables (e.g., grated carrots, tomatoes, cucumber, hearts of palm, broccoli)
- 4-ounce steamed chicken breast
- 2 tablespoons of low-fat vinaigrette
- 1 cup of iced tea

SNACK

- 1 cup raspberries with Greek yogurt
- 1 cup of flavored water

DINNER

- 4-ounce filet mignon
- 1 cup of grilled asparagus
- 1 glass of red wine

DESSERT

- 1 cup of sugar-free Jell-O
- 1 cup of green tea

PERSON THREE: AVERAGE "HEALTHY" DIET

BREAKFAST

- 1 cup of Special K cereal
- 1 cup of skim milk
- 1 banana

LUNCH

- Caesar salad with grilled chicken
- 1 cup of diet iced tea

SNACK

- 1 granola bar

DINNER

- 1 cup of miso soup
- 1 side salad
- 1 spicy tuna roll
- 1 California roll
- 1 cup of green tea

Now ask yourself these questions: Which of these individuals eats the most food? Which person consumes the most calories? How would you rank these diets, from healthiest to least healthy?

You probably guessed that person two's diet ranks the healthiest, but did you know it also provided the most food for the least calories? And you'll be surprised to learn that our person three, who thought she was making healthy choices, isn't that much better off than person one, who is clearly making the least healthy choices.

Here's how they add up:

High-Fiber Diet: The day's food intake for person two adds up to just 1400 calories and delivers a whopping 60 grams of fiber.

Average "Healthy" Eater: Person three's meager menu comes in at 2,306 calories and only 11 grams of fiber, which is less than half the fiber an average woman needs each day and barely one-third of a man's daily requirement. And even with all those calories, she probably still felt hungry and deprived.

Typical American Diet: The menu for person one packs 2,729 calories, yet it lacks in nutrients and has a paltry 10 grams of fiber. Notice how close it is, nutritionally, to the supposedly health-conscious diet. Neither of those two individuals can expect to lose weight with these choices.

WHY FAD DIETS DON'T LAST— AND WHY THE F-FACTOR WAY WILL

Many of my new clients find their way to my office after they've run the gamut of fad diets and their own do-it-yourself weight-loss schemes. Here's the simple truth: You can lose some weight on any diet, whether you're eating cabbage soup or cookies, as long as it creates a caloric deficit and you're consuming fewer calories than you burn each day. It's easy to get excited about the newest magic bullet that promises superquick weight loss. But could you stick to a diet like that for the rest of your life? Of course not.

Diets that severely reduce calories by cutting out food are doomed to fail because they simply aren't sustainable. No one can go very long feeling hungry and deprived, and what happens next is predictable: the dieter gives up and gives in to all of his or her cravings. Whatever weight was lost then comes right back and then some. One of the main reasons people succeed at losing weight the F-Factor way is that it doesn't leave you hungry or longing for all the foods you used to love. You lose weight without sacrificing your lifestyle.

Because you are adding rather than omitting foods to your diet, the Miracle Carb Diet makes it easier not only to take the weight off but also to maintain your ideal weight. If you've dieted before, you probably know how unpleasant it can be—hunger pangs, constipation, headaches, and light-headedness. On the Miracle Carb Diet, you will start looking and feeling better right from the start. Take that familiar late-afternoon slump that sends you to the vending machine or coffee shop like clockwork every day: How long does that pick-me-up really last? Probably not very long if you are eating processed foods with refined carbohydrates, such as cookies or chips. That's because refined carbs cause your blood sugar level to spike and then crash. At first you do get a quick little burst of energy, but in no time you feel tired again—and hungry again.

Eating a lot of refined carbohydrates sets up a cycle of hunger that is driven largely by cravings for a sugar boost. Every time you give in to those cravings, you consume a lot of unnecessary calories that can easily lead to weight gain. But, as you will see, not all carbohydrates are bad for your waistline. The right carbs—especially those high in fiber—are not calorie bombs, nor do they burn quickly or cause blood sugar levels to spike and fall.

Remember my client Stacey? She couldn't figure out why she wasn't losing weight even though she had drastically cut back on calories and eliminated most carbs from her diet.

"Your body doesn't want to waste energy," I explained to her. "It's a sophisticated machine that's designed to help you survive in even the most adverse circumstances. That's why you sometimes hear these stories on the news about lost hikers miraculously going for days without food but being found alive. If you eat too few calories, your body goes into self-preservation mode, thinking there's a food shortage, and your metabolism automatically begins to slow down in order to save as much energy as possible. As far as your body is concerned, a drastic diet signals the same kind of emergency as being lost in the wilderness. Hunger is hunger, and being chronically hungry can make you fat. On the other hand, fiber will satisfy hunger, add bulk without calories to food, and then burn calories as the body works to digest it."

When you eat carbohydrates, whether in the form of starch, fruit, or milk, they get converted into glucose, which is stored in your muscles and liver as glycogen. Glycogen is how your body stores sugar for the short term. The average-size person stores a total of 350 grams of glycogen per day. About 100 grams of that fuel is stored in your liver, and the rest is stored in your muscle. The liver and muscle are like dual fuel tanks. When those tanks reach their capacity, any excess calories from eating starchy carbohydrates cause your glycogen stores to overflow. The trouble is that extra glucose doesn't magically disappear just because the designated storage tanks are full. Your body recognizes it as energy and protectively converts it to fat and stashes it away for later use in case of an emergency, such as famine. There's no limit to the amount of fat the body can store, so the more excess glucose you give it, the fatter you will become. The point I want to emphasize here is that carbohydrates on their own do not make you fat. The excess of what your body can store as glycogen is to blame for that.

That doesn't mean that calories don't count. If your total energy requirement, based on your body type and size, is 1,800 calories, and you eat 2,000 calories per day, it's not going to matter if all 2,000 calories came from lean chicken and steamed veggies: You're still going to gain weight. The only way to lose weight is to take in fewer calories than your body burns. One pound of stored body fat equals approximately 3,500 calories.

From the outset, the Miracle Carb Diet creates a caloric deficit: When the body needs energy, it breaks down glucose first, then fat, and finally protein. Only in the absence of glucose does the body burn fat, and to make this happen the key is to eat foods that fill your glycogen stores, but not to the point of overflowing. This is how the Miracle Carb Diet works to keep you in a fat-burning mode. Other diets eliminate food to create a caloric deficit but in ways that can actually slow metabolism and make it harder to lose weight.

The body burns more calories digesting protein than it does digesting fat or carbohydrates. (It can take as much as 25 percent more energy to digest protein compared to fat.) Adding fiber and lean protein boosts the metabolism in digestion. Healthy sources of protein include lean beef, turkey, fish, white meat chicken, tofu, nuts, beans, eggs, and low-fat dairy products.

On F-Factor's Miracle Carb Diet, you won't be counting calories, though. Your focus instead will be on the amount of fiber you consume—ideally 30–35 grams a day. You'll be eating delicious, nutritious foods that will help fill you up without ever filling you out.

Here's what you can expect as you begin this exciting transformation:

Stage One of the program will jump-start your metabolism by limiting (but not eliminating!) carbohydrates while replacing the refined, processed foods you've been eating with more nutritious, fiber-rich choices. This phase will last about two weeks, and during this time you can expect to lose 6–10 pounds. Stage Two will gradually incorporate more carbs into your daily food plan, so you will be eating more while losing another 4–10 pounds. In about one month, you will reach Stage Three—what I like to call the homestretch. You'll have lost 10–20 pounds or more and be on pace to reach your goal weight. If you are looking to lose about 20 pounds, you can expect to reach your goal weight in about two months. If you have more to lose, you'll stay on Stage Three until you reach your goal, losing at a rate of 1–2 pounds per week. During this time you will be amazed not only by how much slimmer you are but by how radiant you look and feel as your body thrives on all the nutrients it's getting. Stage Four is the final maintenance phase that will be your "new normal" for healthy living. Old, unhealthy habits will be history, and so will cravings and the frustration you felt about your weight.

Now let's get started!

WAYS FIBER HELPS YOU FEEL
AND LOOK YOUR BEST

More Energy

Combining fiber and lean protein at every meal and at snack time keeps blood glucose levels steady, providing your body with sustained energy. Eating refined carbohydrates creates spikes in blood sugar, producing a fast energy rush followed by sudden drop that can leave you feeling tired and craving more refined carbs to get your sugar level back up.

Flatter Stomach

Eating a high-fiber diet helps you have complete and regular bowel movements. Fiber increases stool bulk, which helps prevent constipation. The Miracle Carb Diet eliminates bloating and can offer relief from irritable bowel syndrome.

Clearer Skin

Fiber soaks up toxins in the blood and eliminates them through the digestive tract instead of your pores, leading to brighter, clearer skin. Plus fruits and vegetables are rich in antioxidants that fight aging.

Improved Sleep

Eating refined carbs late in the day causes your blood sugar level to peak and then crash during sleep, which is why some people get up to eat something in the middle of the night. Eating food rich in fiber helps keep blood sugars steady, which in turn helps you wake up feeling rested.

HEALTH BENEFITS OF EATING FIBER

If you saw a food label that said, "May reduce the risk of heart disease, diabetes, and cancer; lower your cholesterol; and control your appetite," you might think it was a scam. Yet that is exactly what fiber does. Adding fiber-rich foods to your diet is one of the best things you can do to increase your chances for a long and healthy life.

Protect against Heart Disease and Stroke

Cardiovascular disease (CVD) is the single leading cause of death in the United States, and more than 70 million Americans have it in some form. A good gauge of a person's heart health is blood lipids—HDL and LDL cholesterol as well as triglycerides; the lower your LDL and triglyceride levels, the less likely you are to develop CVD. Many Americans take cholesterol-lowering medications, such as statins, but dietary changes can be effective as well, and the best change of all is to eat more fiber. Fiber helps to lower cholesterol by absorbing cholesterol in the gastrointestinal tract and moving it out of the body before it can reach the bloodstream and clog up arteries. Hundreds of my clients have made remarkable improvements in their cholesterol levels in as little as eight weeks, and many who were taking statin drugs were able to lower their dosage or even discontinue their medication.

Lower Diabetes Risk

Diabetes is growing at an alarming rate in the United States. According to the American Diabetes Association, 25.8 million adults and children in America have diabetes and another 79 million have prediabetes. People with prediabetes can delay or prevent diabetes through lifestyle changes that include diet, weight loss, and exercise. The Miracle Carb Diet can be highly effective because not only will it produce weight loss, but eating fiber and lean protein also helps stabilize blood sugar levels throughout the day. Research has shown that by eating a high-fiber diet, people can lower their risk of diabetes by 30 percent.[1]

---

1. Franz, Marion J., John M. Bantle, Christine A. Beebe, et al. "American Diabetes Association Position Statement: Evidence-Based Nutrition Principles and Recommendations for the Treatment and Prevention of Diabetes and Related Complications," *Journal of the American Dietetic Association* 102, no. 1 (Jan. 2002): 109–118.

Reduces the Risk for Breast Cancer

Breast cancer among women has risen from 1 in 20 in 1960 to 1 in 8 today, making it the leading cancer among white and African American women. Studies have found a strong correlation between eating a diet that is high in fiber and reduced breast cancer risk. One study reported in the *Journal of Clinical Oncology* found that a diet with 20–30 grams of fiber per day can lower blood estrogen levels. Estrogen is a factor in the early growth and development of breast cancer, and lowering estrogen levels in the body may lower your risk. There are several theories about how dietary fiber helps lower estrogen levels. One theory is that fiber interferes with the absorption of estrogen into the blood. Another theory is that people who eat more fiber may consume less fat, and a diet that is high in fat is believed to increase the risk of developing breast cancer.

Lower Blood Pressure

About one in five Americans have high blood pressure, which is defined as blood pressure above 140/90. It's estimated that 50 percent of people between the ages of fifty-five and sixty-five have high blood pressure—also known as hypertension—and, if left unchecked, it can lead to stroke, heart failure, heart attack, and death. One way to address high blood pressure is by eating more fiber, which reduces insulin resistance and helps with weight control—each a factor in hypertension risk.

Protect against Colon Cancer

Not including skin cancers, colon cancer is the third most common cancer in men and women in the United States and the second leading cause of cancer-related deaths. Studies have found diets high in fiber (30 grams or more fiber per day) lower the risk of colon cancer by 40 percent. It is believed that fiber fights colon cancer by binding to carcinogens in the gut and quickly eliminating them through the colon.

Alleviate Constipation

Constipation is one of the most common gastrointestinal complaints, and by definition it means having less than three bowel movements per week. Many people turn to laxatives, but overuse can cause damage to the intestines and colon and actually make constipation worse. Getting more dietary fiber through the foods you eat is the best way to prevent or alleviate consipation. Simply put, fiber adds bulk to stool, and this allows for easy, regular defecation. The Miracle Carb Diet, with its 35 grams of fiber a day coming from fruits and vegetables, promises to alleviate constipation once and for all.

THE MIRACLE CARB DIET

Now that you understand the philosophy and the science behind the F-Factor way, you're ready to begin the diet itself. The Miracle Carb plan is built around four separate stages, each one designed to take fullest advantage of the positive changes you're going to experience in your metabolism, so you can maximize your weight loss as effortlessly as possible.

Before you start, be sure to check out the sidebar below on reading food labels, so you understand how to easily calculate the net carbohydrates per serving in any food you're picking up at the grocery store, whether it's an old favorite or something new you're trying. You won't need any special scales or calorie counters on the Miracle Carb Diet, and you won't need to decipher mystery ingredients. The Miracle Carb Bible at the back of this book provides the serving size and nutritional information you need for all foods, beverages, and condiments in the diet.

READING FOOD LABELS

Throughout my years in private practice, nearly all of my new clients come in as frustrated calorie counters. They are amazed—even skeptical—when I tell them that we don't count calories. While calories are important, even more important are two numbers found on the Nutrition Facts label of food products: Total Carbohydrate and Dietary Fiber.

First of all, fiber makes calories disappear! Fiber is the indigestible part of the carbohydrate, and the more fiber a food has, the fewer net carbohydrates it contains. Fiber cannot be digested, which means it has zero calories. The fiber passes through the digestive tract and exits the body, so there's no reason to count it. Only the carb portion of the food goes to the muscle and liver stores.

Starting on Stage One, you'll be choosing foods based on their net carbs, and you will track net carbs in your daily journal. It's simple to calculate net carbs. Refer to the Nutrition Facts label of any food product (or for whole foods, refer to the Miracle Carb Bible in the appendix section) and note the values per serving for Dietary Fiber and Total Carbohydrate. Subtract the Dietary Fiber from the Total Carbohydrate and the result gives you your net carbohydrate.

$$\text{Total Carbohydrate} - \text{Dietary Fiber} = \text{Net Carbohydrate}$$

Here's how to calculate the net carbs for two different food labels.

Example: Nature's Own Wheat Bread vs. Pepperidge Farm White Bread

NATURE'S OWN 40-CALORIE WHEAT

Nutrition Facts
Serving Size: 2 slices

Amount per serving	
Calories 80	Calories from Fat 5
	%Daily Value*
Total Fat 0.5 g	1%
Saturated Fat 0 g	0%
Trans Fat 0 g	
Cholestrol 0 mg	0%
Sodium 100 mg	7%
Total Carbohydrate 20 g	7%
Dietary Fiber 6 g	23%
Sugars 1 g	
Protein 5 g	

*%Daily values (DV) are based on a 2,000 calorie diet

PEPPERIDGE FARM® WHITE SANDWICH BREAD

Nutrition Facts
Serving Size: 2 slices

Amount per serving	
Calories 130	Calories from Fat 20
	%Daily Value*
Total Fat 2.5 g	4%
Saturated Fat 0.5 g	2%
Trans Fat 0 g	
Cholestrol 0 mg	0%
Sodium 230 mg	10%
Total Carbohydrate 23 g	8%
Dietary Fiber <1g	4%
Sugars 3g	
Protein 4g	

*%Daily values (DV) are based on a 2,000 calorie diet

Nature's Own 40-Calorie Wheat Bread has 10 grams of carbohydrate and 3 grams of fiber per slice. To determine the net carbohydrate, you subtract the fiber from the total carbohydrate listed on the label.

10 grams carbohydrate – 3 grams fiber = 7 grams net carbohydrate

So if you're eating a slice of Nature's Own for a bread serving on the Miracle Carb plan, you count it as 7 grams of carbohydrate.

By comparison, the same serving of Pepperidge Farm White Sandwich Bread (1 slice) contains 11.5 grams of carbohydrate and less than .5 gram of fiber.

11.5 grams carbohydrate – .5 gram fiber = 11 grams net carbohydrate

You are getting 4 grams more net carbohydrate from the white bread than from the wheat bread.

Not only does the wheat bread contain less net carbohydrate than the white bread, but it also contains fewer calories. That's true across the board: The more fiber in a food, the fewer calories it will contain. You can have double the portion size of the Nature's Own 40 Calorie Wheat Bread (80 calories for 2 slices) as compared to the white bread.

I've included answers to the most frequently asked questions my clients have at each stage, and at the end of the book, you'll find my best recipes for eating the F-Factor way, whether you're just starting the diet or are enjoying your new lifestyle after achieving your goal weight. Get ready to truly savor your success!

On the Miracle Carb Diet, all animal proteins such as chicken, beef, fish, and eggs are journaled as 0 grams of carbohydrate and 0 grams of fiber. The same is true for cheese, Greek yogurt, tofu, and other soy products. Even though you may see on the nutrition label that your Greek yogurt contains some grams of carbohydrate, because there is far more protein than there are carbs, it is considered a protein.

STAGE ONE: REV UP YOUR METABOLISM

Duration: 2 weeks

Focus: Incorporate these three permitted high-fiber carbs and eliminate all others:

- ☞ High-fiber crackers
- ☞ High-fiber cereal
- ☞ Fruit

Total Net Carb: 35 grams per day

Total Fiber Goal: 35 grams or more per day

What to Expect: 6–10 pounds weight loss

Stage One is about getting your engine going—we're going to rev up your metabolism by adding fiber-rich foods to your diet and scaling back your use of refined, processed food. On Stage One, you'll eat three servings of carbohydrate a day: a serving of high-fiber cereal, a serving of fresh fruit, and a minimum of four high-fiber crackers (with at least 5 grams of fiber per serving). You will also eat plenty of lean protein, such as chicken, fish, beef, Greek yogurt, and cheese; as many non-starchy vegetables as you like; and some heart-healthy fat. You can even enjoy wine and spirits in moderation.

By eliminating all the refined carbohydrates from your diet, Stage One allows you to start with a clean slate. This keeps things nice and simple. The reason I chose these three carbohydrates for Stage One is that they are high in fiber; they fill you up by adding bulk and volume, yet they are naturally low in calories and fat. Limiting your choices for the next two weeks will also help you realize just how many carbohydrates you were eating before.

During this stage, you will begin tracking what you eat in a daily journal using the simple chart provided in this chapter. Filling in the journal not only makes you accountable for what you eat, but it also teaches you how the foods you choose work toward meeting your daily fiber goals. On the Miracle Carb Diet, you maximize your weight loss by knowing not only which foods to eat but also which ones to combine. You'll learn that eating fiber and protein at every meal makes losing weight no big deal.

By carefully following the program as outlined in this chapter, you can expect to lose between 6–10 pounds during this initial two-week period. You are likely to notice other benefits as well: clearer skin, a better night's sleep, and an ability to stay more focused and alert during the day. Most of my new clients marvel at how much more energy they have. Women and men alike say they no longer feel bloated and notice that their tummy is flatter. By adding the Miracle Carb to your diet, I guarantee you will never feel hungry or deprived again and—finally—losing weight will seem effortless.

CARBOHYDRATES PERMITTED
ON STAGE ONE

On the Miracle Carb Diet, 15 grams is considered a single serving of carbohydrate. This amount is based on established standards from the Dietary Exchange List that includes starches, fruits and juices, milks and yogurts—all are similar in nutrient content and so have been designated as 15 grams of carbohydrate servings.

During Stage One, you are permitted three specific carbohydrates each day:

- 1 serving of any cereal with 20–25 grams of carbohydrate and 12–13 grams of fiber per serving
- A minimum of four high-fiber crackers, containing at least 5 grams of fiber and no more than 2 grams of net carbohydrate per serving
- 1 serving of fruit

NON-STARCHY VEGETABLES

From day one, you can have as many non-starchy vegetables as you want. Non-starchy vegetables like asparagus, beets, cabbage, broccoli, hearts of palm, and salad greens are high-fiber carbs with only 25 calories and 5 grams of carbs per serving. Because the calories and carbs are so low and they are high in fiber, journal these as 0 grams of carbs and refer to the Miracle Carb Bible for their fiber content. For example, a half cup of cooked broccoli would be journaled as 0 grams of carbs and 2 grams of fiber. Non-starchy vegetables are free foods, packed with fiber, vitamins, minerals, and antioxidants, and you can fill up on them as you like as long as they are raw or steamed. Don't prepare them with oil or butter, which won't add carbs but will add a lot of calories from fat.

LEAN PROTEIN

Adding lean protein in combination with fiber at every meal and snack will keep you feeling full and satisfied. Protien is essential for building lean muscle mass, and adding muscle boosts metabolism and also makes room to store more carbs in the future. Check out Tanya's Toppers on page 48—my simple, delicious protein toppings that go perfectly with high-fiber crackers. When journaling, proteins are counted as 0 grams of carbs and 0 grams of fiber.

On Stage One, you should have protein throughout the day:

Breakfast: 4–6 ounces
Lunch: 4–6 ounces
Snack: 2–4 ounces
Dinner: 4–6 ounces

FATS

We need some fat in our diet for transporting vitamins and normal body function. A little bit of fat at each meal is okay because it slows down digestion and keeps you feeling fuller a bit longer. Choose heart-healthy monounsaturated fats such as olive oil, avocado, and nuts (e.g., pistachios). Though fats are journaled as 0 grams of *carbohydrate*, remember that even a small amount can still add a lot of *calories*. Let me emphasize that fats are *not* a free food: 1 tablespoon of oil or butter contains 135 calories and 15 grams of fat, and that can easily lead to weight gain. Be especially careful when dining out, because that's when it's easy to add fats to your food.

BEVERAGES

It is important to drink 3 liters (approximately 12 cups) of water per day. When people start the diet, they can feel bloated, distended, or constipated if, like most Americans, they're not drinking sufficient water. Water helps soften fiber so it can easily pass through the gastrointestinal system and work its magic by absorbing fat, calories from other foods, cholesterol, estrogen, and other toxins and ushering them out of the body.

Being dehydrated can also mimic hunger. Many times, our hunger is really just thirst in disguise, making us feel weak, cranky, and tired. It's tempting to grab a candy bar, but to get rid of these symptoms all we really need is a drink of zero-calorie water. You might find it easier to get enough water if you add a calorie-free flavor enhancer. Feel free to include unsweetened beverages such as diet soda, coffee, tea, and vegetable juice in your daily plan, but they are not substitutes for water. For guidelines on drinking alcohol see Chapter 6: Raise Your Glass.

STAGE ONE SHOPPING LIST

If your diet has been lacking in fiber, Stage One will gently introduce high-fiber foods to your digestive system. In time, you will be enjoying fiber in its many varieties. Adding too much fiber too soon can cause discomfort, so don't get overzealous. For the next two weeks you'll eat just enough fiber to rev up your metabolism while allowing your body to get accustomed to it.

Here's what you can add to your shopping cart for Stage One:

Carbs

→ High-fiber crackers containing no more than 25 calories and at least 5 grams of fiber per cracker
→ High-fiber cereal (one serving of any cereal with 20–25 grams of carbs and 12–13 grams of fiber per serving)
→ Fruits

Vegetables

→ See the Miracle Carb Bible on page 316 for the highest-fiber veggies

Yogurt and Eggs

→ 0% Greek yogurt, plain
→ Fage Total 0% Yogurt
→ Chobani Yogurt
→ Stonyfield Farm Oikos Organic Greek Yogurt
→ Eggland's Best Eggs
→ Eggology 100% Egg Whites

Cheese (with 0–3 grams of fat per ounce)

→ Laughing Cow Light Wedges (all flavors)
→ Kraft Natural Cheese Fat Free Slices and Shredded

→ Mini Babybel Light

→ Athenos Reduced Fat Traditional Feta Cheese

→ Friendship Farmer Cheese

→ Part skim string cheese

→ Fat-free or part skim ricotta

→ Parmesan cheese

→ Light n' Lively Lowfat Cottage Cheese

→ Friendship 1% Lowfat Cottage Cheese

→ Axelrod Lowfat Cottage Cheese

Deli Meats (with 0–3 grams of fat per ounce)

→ Sliced turkey breast (white meat)

→ Sliced chicken breast (white meat)

→ Sliced roast beef

→ Sliced ham

Fish (fresh or frozen) (with 0–3 grams of fat per ounce)

→ Salmon (fresh or canned)

→ Tuna (fresh or canned in water or StarKist Flavor Fresh Pouch
   tuna in water)

→ Catfish

→ Cod

→ Flounder

→ Haddock

→ Halibut

→ Herring (uncreamed or smoked)

→ Smoked salmon

→ Sardines

→ Sole

→ Snapper

→ Trout

Shellfish (fresh or frozen) (with 0–3 grams of fat per ounce)

→ Clams

→ Crab

→ Lobster

→ Scallops

→ Shrimp

→ Squid

→ Oysters

→ Mussels

Pork (with 0–3 grams of fat per ounce)

→ Ham lean (canned, smoked, or boiled)

→ Canadian bacon

→ Tenderloin

→ Center loin chop

Poultry (with 0–3 grams of fat per ounce)

→ Chicken or turkey (white meat, no skin)

→ Ground chicken or turkey breast

→ Turkey bacon

→ Chicken or turkey lean sausage

→ Cornish hen

→ Applegate Farms Organic Turkey Hot Dogs

Beef (with 0–3 grams of fat per ounce)

→ Lean beef (< 90%)

→ Round

→ Sirloin

→ Flank steak

→ Tenderloin

→ Roast (rib, chuck, rump)

- → Steak (T-bone, porterhouse, cubed)
- → Ground round

Lamb/Veal (with 0–3 grams of fat per ounce)

- → Lamb (roast, chop, leg)
- → Veal (chop, leg)
- → Duck or pheasant (skinless)
- → Venison
- → Buffalo

Dessert

- → Sugar-Free Jell-O
- → Tofutti Chocolate Fudge Treats
- → Swiss Miss Sensible Sweets Diet Cocoa (25 calories)
- → Attune Chocolate Probiotic Bar
- → No-sugar-added Popsicle

Cooking Sprays

- → Nonstick cooking spray

Condiments

- → Balsamic vinegar
- → Salsa
- → Lemon or lime juice
- → Wish-Bone Salad Spritzers or Ken's Lite Dressings
- → Mustard
- → Tomato sauce (Rao's or Healthy Choice)
- → Nonnutritive sweetener
- → Sugar-free jelly (Polaner Sugar Free with Fiber)

Nuts
→ Pistachios
→ Peanuts
→ Almonds
→ Walnuts
→ Pecans
→ Bell Plantation PB2 (powdered peanut butter substitute; see sidebar on page 60)

HOW TO JOURNAL

As you start Stage One, make enough copies of the journal grid to last for two weeks, including a few spares in case you need them. Alternatively, you will find printable journal grids for Stages One, Two, and Three at FFactor.com.

Enter your food choices for every meal and for the snacks you eat each day. On the right-hand side of the journal you'll enter your carb and fiber totals for each food item. If you can't find those totals in the Miracle Carb Bible, look for them on your food labels.

At the end of the day, add up all the carbohydrates and put the total above the letter *A* at the bottom of the left column.

Next, add up the fiber grams and put the total above the letter *B* in the bottom-right column.

Finally, subtract the total fiber from the total carbohydrate to get your net carbohydrate for the day.

A (total carbohydrate) − B (total fiber) = C (net carbohydrate)

Write the net carbohydrate in the circle.

Review your daily journal entries to check . . .

Miracle Carb Diet Journal

DATE	CARB (A)	FIBER (B)
BREAKFAST		
LUNCH		
SNACK		
DINNER		
DESSERT		
TOTAL		

A – B = C

Total Carb	Total Fiber	Net Carb

◯

A

B > 30

<35 g NET CARB

- Did you meet your fiber goal for the day?
- Did you stay below 35 grams net carbohydrate?
- Did you eat every meal and snack?
- Did you have a serving of fruit?
- Did you stay well hydrated?

WHY KEEP A JOURNAL?

Journaling is important for many reasons. First and foremost, journaling makes you accountable. Even if it's "just a few" jelly beans you're grabbing from your officemate's bowl on your way to the elevator, consistently writing down what you put in your mouth keeps you honest and that much more inclined to stay the course.

By sticking to the diet and journaling each day, you can't help but lose weight. Without keeping a journal, especially during Stage One, you're leaving yourself vulnerable to careless mistakes that you would otherwise catch at the outset. The bottom line is that journaling provides you with the framework for success.

Don't worry about the week, the month, or the future. Using your journal, just take it one day at a time. Focus on following through today, and your success will grow incrementally.

SAMPLE DAY

Breakfast
⅓ cup of Kellogg's All-Bran Bran Buds
1 cup of 0% plain Greek yogurt
1¼ cups of sliced strawberries
Coffee with 2 tablespoons of fat-free half-and-half and
nonnutritive sweetener

On Stage One your net carb goal is 35 grams or less. On Stage Two, your goal will be 45 grams. On Stage Three, you'll be averaging about 65 grams net carbs each day. As you can see, you will be eating more net carbs as you continue to lose weight. Your daily fiber goal remains the same throughout the diet—at least 35 grams.

Lunch

Large salad with mixed non-starchy vegetables (e.g., broccoli, carrots, tomatoes, cucumber, hearts of palm)
F-Factor Vinaigrette (balsamic vinegar plus 2 tablespoons of grated Parmesan)
1 cup chicken and vegetable soup
Water or diet soda

Snack

F-Factor Pizza (4 high-fiber crackers topped with ¼ cup of 1% cottage cheese,
2 tablespoons of tomato sauce, and 1 tablespoon of Parmesan cheese)
Unsweetened iced tea

Dinner

Small chopped salad with F-Factor Vinaigrette
4-ounce Steamed "Miso-Glazed" Cod (recipe on page 203)
½ cup of roasted artichoke hearts
1 glass of wine

Dessert

Lemonade Popsicle (recipe on page 214)
Decaffeinated coffee

SAMPLE STAGE ONE JOURNAL

DATE	CARB (A)	FIBER (B)
BREAKFAST		
⅓ cup Kellogg's All-Bran Bran Buds	24	13
1 cup 0% plain Greek yogurt	0	0
1¼ cups sliced strawberries	15	4
Coffee	0	0
LUNCH		
Large salad with mixed non-starchy vegetables (broccoli, carrots, tomatoes, hearts of palm, cucumber, etc.)	0	6
F-Factor Vinaigrette (balsamic vinegar plus 2 tablespoons grated Parmesan cheese)	0	0
1 cup chicken and vegetable soup	0	3
Water or diet soda	0	0
SNACK		
F-Factor Pizza (4 high-fiber crackers topped with ¼ cup of 1% cottage cheese, 2 tablespoons of tomato sauce, and 1 tablespoon of Parmesan cheese)	28	20
Unsweetened iced tea	0	0
DINNER		
Small chopped salad with F-Factor Vinaigrette	0	3
4-ounce Steamed "Miso-Glazed" Cod	0	3
½ cup roasted artichoke hearts	0	4
1 glass wine	2	0
DESSERT		
Lemonade Popsicle	0	0
Decaffeinated coffee	0	0
TOTAL	69	56

A – B = C

Total Carb	Total Fiber	Net Carb

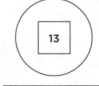

13

<35 g NET CARB

A

B > 30

CHEAT SHEET: JOURNALING ON STAGE ONE

Here's a quick-glance list to help you get started with journaling. Most of the foods on Stage One can be found here.

	Carbohydrate	Fiber
CEREAL		
½ cup Fiber One	25 grams	14 grams
½ cup All Bran, Extra Fiber	20 grams	13 grams
⅓ cup All-Bran Bran Buds	24 grams	13 grams
All other cereals (containing 20–25 grams carbs and 12–13 grams fiber)	See Miracle Carb Bible	See Miracle Carb Bible
OTHER FOODS		
Fruit	15 grams	See Miracle Carb Bible
High-fiber crackers (per cracker)	7 grams	5 grams
Non-starchy vegetables	0 grams	See Miracle Carb Bible
Large salad with veggies	0 grams	~6 grams
Small appetizer salad	0 grams	~3 grams
PROTEIN (AIM FOR LEAN PROTEINS WITH 0-3 GRAMS OF FAT PER OUNCE)		
Poultry, fish, beef/veal/pork, PB2, tofu, cheese/1% cottage cheese/fat-free plain Greek yogurt	0 grams	0 grams
CONDIMENTS		
Mustard, F-Factor Vinaigrette, soy sauce, cocktail sauce, low-fat mayonnaise, etc.	0 grams	0 grams

(continued)

	Carbohydrate	Fiber
ALCOHOL		
Wine (5-ounce glass)	2 grams	0 grams
Spirits (1 ounce)	0 grams	0 grams
Beer/cocktails	15 grams	0 grams
FATS (USE SPARINGLY)		
Olive oil, cream cheese, avocado, nuts/nut butters, margarine, butter, etc.	0 g	0 g
Desserts in Stage One	0 g	0 g

STAGE ONE MENU CHOICES

Net Carb: 35 grams or less per day

Breakfast (choose one of the following):

1) High-fiber crackers with Tanya's Toppers
   4 High-fiber crackers with Tanya's Toppers (breakfast choices)
   Optional: 1 serving of fruit

2) F-Factor Fruit and Yogurt Cereal Parfait
   ½ cup of Fiber One, or ⅓ cup of Bran Buds cereal or other high-fiber cereal
   ½–1 cup of 1% cottage cheese, or nonfat plain Greek yogurt (Fage, Chobani, Oikos, etc.)
   Optional: 1 serving of fruit, 1 teaspoon (packet) nonnutritive sweetener, cinnamon to taste

3) F-Factor Smoothie

    6-ounce cup of Greek yogurt (Fage Total 0% Yogurt, Chobani, etc.)

    $3/4$ cup of frozen berries (raspberries, blueberries, strawberries)

    $1/5$ frozen banana

    $1/2$ cup of Fiber One Original

    1–3 tablespoons of water

    Optional: 1 teaspoon (packet) nonnutritive sweetener

Tip: *Cut the banana into small pieces, wrap in Saran wrap, and freeze for an hour.*

4) Hot Cereal—"Morning Glory" plus Protein

    Mix the ingredients listed below. Stir to an oatmeal-like consistency.

    $1/2$ cup of cracker crumbs (3 high-fiber crackers, crushed)

    $1/4$ cup of Fiber One Original

    2 tablespoons of PB2

    2 teaspoons of nonnutritive sweetener

    $1/4$ teaspoon of cinnamon

    $1/4$–$1/2$ cup of hot water

    Optional: 1 serving of fruit

Add a protein: You must use some of your daily protein allowance here by adding 6 ounces of Greek yogurt, or 3–4 egg whites, or $1/2$ cup of cottage cheese, or 2 tablespoons of protein powder mixed into the "Morning Glory."

Beverage options: Tea or coffee with 1–2 tablespoons of fat-free half-and-half and a nonnutritive sweetener, tomato juice/V8, or water

Lunch (choose one of the following):

1) F-Factor Salad plus Protein

    Salad (use mixed greens, spinach, or romaine as your bulk with non-starchy vegetables)

Lean protein (4–6 ounces)

F-Factor Vinaigrette (mix vinegar with mustard or Parmesan cheese) or Wish-Bone Salad Spritzer/Walden Farms dressing

2) Protein and Veggies

Lean protein (4–6 ounces)

Non-starchy vegetable

Note: *When a vegetable is steamed without any oil, or prepared using a nonstick cooking spray, you can eat the whole portion. However, if it is sautéed, grilled, or broiled in oil, eat half the portion.*

3) High-fiber crackers and Tanya's Toppers with Salad, Veggies, or Soup

Side salad/non-starchy vegetables or 1 cup of soup (e.g., a broth-based soup such as gazpacho, chicken/vegetable, miso, or consommé)

4) High-fiber crackers with Tanya's Toppers (lunch choices)

Beverage options: Water, sugar-free beverages, tomato juice/V8, tea, or coffee

Snack:

1) High-fiber crackers and Tanya's Toppers

4 high-fiber crackers with Tanya's Toppers (snack choices)

2) F-Factor Fruit and Yogurt Cereal Parfait

3) F-Factor Smoothies

Beverage options: Water, sugar-free beverages (such as Diet Snapple), tomato juice/V8, iced or hot tea, or coffee.

Dinner:

Entrée (choose one of the following):

1) Soup or Salad with a Protein Appetizer and Non-Starchy Vegetables
    Soup or salad
    Protein-based appetizer
    Non-starchy vegetable

2) Salad and an Entrée and Non-Starchy Vegetables
    Lean protein (women: 3–4 ounces protein, men: 6–8 ounces protein)
    Non-starchy vegetable

Note: *Women eat half the protein served in a restaurant; men eat ⅔ of the protein served, even if it's fish or chicken.*

Beverage options: Water, wine, or spirits

Dessert (choose one of the following):

1) Sugar-Free Jell-O with Sugar-Free Fat-Free Whipped Cream

2) Sugar-Free Diet Hot Chocolate (Swiss Miss Sensible Sweets Diet Cocoa, 25 calories)

3) 1 Tofutti Chocolate Fudge Treat, Fudgsicle, or Creamsicle (no sugar added)

4) Small Serving of Fruit (if you have not already had your fruit serving)

5) Arctic Zero Frozen Desserts (½ cup serving)

Beverage options: Decaffeinated, unsweetened hot or iced tea or coffee, water

TANYA'S TOPPERS

There are so many ways to pair fiber and protein. Start with a high-fiber cracker and try any of these tasty toppers:

Breakfast Toppers:

→ 4–6 egg whites (scrambled, hard-boiled, or as an omelet) made with your favorite vegetables and 1–2 Laughing Cow Light cheese wedges or low-fat cheese

→ 2–4 slices of lox with 2 Laughing Cow Light cheese wedges or low-fat/ nonfat cream cheese (optional: onion and tomato)

→ ½–1 cup of low-fat cottage cheese or 4–6 ounces nonfat plain Greek yogurt. For a sweet bite, use a packet of Splenda and cinnamon to taste. For a savory flavor, spread the cottage cheese or yogurt on the crackers and top with tomato slices.

→ 4–6 tablespoons PB2 and 1 tablespoon sugar-free jelly (such as Smucker's or Polaner)

Lunch Toppers:

→ F-Factor Pizza made with ½–1 cup of 1% cottage cheese or low-fat mozzarella, spicy roasted red pepper sauce (such as Lutenica) or tomato sauce, and sprinkle of Parmesan cheese and oregano to taste, and microwaved 1–2 minutes

→ 6 ounces of turkey bacon, chicken, turkey breast, roast beef, or ham (optional: lettuce, tomato, mustard, and Peter Luger Steak House sauce)

→ 2–4 slices of lox with 1–2 Laughing Cow Light cheese wedges or low-fat/ nonfat cream cheese (optional: onion and tomato)

→ ½–1 cup of tuna, egg, or chicken salad (made with low-fat mayonnaise) with lettuce and tomato

Snack Toppers:

→ F-Factor Pizza made with ¼ cup of 1% cottage cheese or low-fat mozzarella, spicy roasted red pepper sauce (such as Lutenica) or tomato sauce, and sprinkle of Parmesan cheese and oregano to taste, and microwaved 1–2 minutes

→ 2–4 slices of lox with 1–2 Laughing Cow Light cheese wedges or low-fat/nonfat cream cheese (optional: onion and tomato)

→ ½ cup of tuna, egg, or chicken salad (made with low-fat mayonnaise)

→ 2–4 ounces of turkey bacon, chicken, turkey breast, roast beef, or ham (optional: lettuce, tomato, mustard, and Peter Luger Steak House sauce)

→ 2–4 Laughing Cow Light cheese wedges with either sugar-free jelly or, for a savory flavor, topped with tomato slices

→ 2–4 tablespoons of PB2 and 1 tablespoon of sugar-free jelly

→ ½ cup of 1% cottage cheese

→ ½ serving of the French Onion/Veggie Dip—Mix two 6 ounce containers fat-free plain Greek yogurt, ½ packet each of onion dip mix and vegetable soup mix, 1 tablespoon low-fat mayo, 1–2 tablespoons of water, and 1 box frozen chopped spinach (first defrost it and then squeeze dry with a paper towel).

THINGS TO REMEMBER

You must eat three full meals and one snack every day. Skipping them does not make the diet work faster; the idea is to eat every three to four hours, which keeps your blood sugar even and prevents hunger and cravings. Going long periods without food will actually stall your weight loss because the body interprets lack of food as reason to store rather than burn calories. The mentality in the United States is to skip breakfast, have a small lunch, then skip snacks to save more room for dinner. We could not have gotten it more wrong! It's important to have a hearty snack because it is an opportunity to get more fiber in and to keep you feeling full so you don't overeat at dinner. As the old adage goes: Eat breakfast like a king, lunch like a prince, and dinner like a pauper. Dinner should be the smallest meal of the day, yet this is typically when people consume the most calories. An average dinner at a restaurant can be anywhere from 2,000–3,000 calories. Think about it: Between the bread basket, appetizer, entrée with sides, and dessert, you're looking at more than a day's worth of calories at one sitting.

"Fiber and protein at every meal makes losing weight no big deal." These are the two nutrients that take the longest time to digest. They help keep you full longer and prevent snacking in between.

Take a multivitamin. During Stage One, I recommend taking a multi-vitamin. Keep in mind that vitamins and supplements are just that. They should not be replacing the foods in your diet. You want to try to get all your vitamins and nutrients from foods first.

FREQUENTLY ASKED QUESTIONS

Am I Getting the Right Crackers?

A high-fiber cracker has at least 5 grams of fiber and no more than 2 net carbs. You calculate net carbs by subtracting a food's dietary fiber content from the total carbs. So, a cracker with 5 grams fiber and 7 grams carbs has 2 net carbs, and counts as a high-fiber cracker. Crackers that meet this criteria work well on the Miracle Carb Diet because, being ultra-high in fiber, they fill you up on very few calories. High-fiber crackers will provide the crunch and variety we want and the fiber boost that we need. See my website, ffactor.com, for specific suitable cracker brands and other Miracle Carb-approved foods.

Can I drink alcohol on Stage One?

Yes, women can have one serving of alcohol per day and men can have two. One of the many reasons the Miracle Carb Diet is so popular and clients are so successful is that you never have to sacrifice your lifestyle or feel that you are giving up your social life. Wine and spirits contain very few calories. If you enjoy a drink, have it. I don't want you to feel deprived, and on the Miracle Carb Diet you won't be.

Why is regular yogurt listed as a carbohydrate while Greek-style yogurt is listed as a non-carbohydrate?

The reason lies in the nutritional content of each yogurt. Six ounces of fat-free yogurt has 15 grams of carbohydrate and only 6 grams of protein. The same 6-ounce serving of Greek-style yogurt has only 7 grams of carbohydrate and 18 grams of protein. Therefore, because Greek-style yogurt has so much more protein than it does carbohydrate, it is listed as a protein source and journaled as 0 grams of carbohydrate and 0 grams of fiber. I love using Greek yogurt as a replacement for milk with cereal. It provides protein and loads of calcium but contains very few calories and carbohydrates. It's also great to use in savory dips and spreads.

I've heard that agave and honey are supposed to be better because they are all natural. Why aren't they on Stage One? And what's the difference between the two?

Agave and honey are natural, but that doesn't mean they are carb- or calorie-free. A tablespoon of either agave or honey contains 70 calories and 17 grams of carbohydrate—that's more carbohydrate than a slice of white bread. Remember, excess carbs get converted into fat, so agave and honey easily add extra carbs and can definitely hinder your efforts to lose weight.

Can I dine out?

Yes, you can dine out even on Stage One. I never want you to put your life on hold just because you are trying to lose weight. There are always healthy choices on a menu. F-Factor is about losing weight while enjoying your life. It's not about turning you into a recluse who has to sit at home eating a mini-size frozen dinner night after night.

Why are ketchup and tomato sauce allowed? I heard they have lots of sugar. Will I gain weight from using them?

Ketchup and tomato sauce are perfectly fine to have even on Stage One. While they do contain some calories and carbs, think about what the real problem at hand is: What do you typically eat with ketchup? French fries? A hamburger? So is it the ketchup or the burger and fries causing you to gain weight? The same can be said about tomato sauce. Is it the big bowl of pasta or the tomato sauce that's the issue? Condiments are generally used sparingly because they pack so much flavor, so not much is needed. Most condiments, such as mustard, soy sauce, and vinegar, contain very few calories and little to no carbs.

STAGE TWO: EAT MORE, BURN MORE

Duration: 2 weeks
Focus: Add one serving of either:

☞ Fruit
☞ Beans, peas, or lentils

Total Net Carb: 45 grams per day
Total Fiber Goal: 35 grams or more per day
What to Expect: 4–10 pounds weight loss

Congratulations! You have successfully made it through Stage One and are well on your way to the top of that mountain! You've made it through the most challenging part, and I can promise you it only gets better from here. By now, you have dropped 6–10 pounds and you are seeing true progress in the way you look and feel. After two weeks following Stage One, you've eliminated many toxins in your body by adding more fiber, and you're no longer feeling bloated, sluggish, or foggy. Your cravings for carbohydrates have decreased significantly, because adding in fiber and protein at every meal has kept your blood glucose levels steady, warding off that all-too-familiar three o'clock slump. The office vending machine has lost its magnetic pull on you, and cookies are no longer considered a staple on your grocery list. Victory is at hand!

You will be on Stage Two for the next two weeks. During this time, you will continue to lose weight and see further improvements resulting from your healthier diet, which is now rich in fiber, vitamins, and antioxidants.

During Stage Two, you will be eating more by adding an extra serving of fruit or a serving from the beans, peas, and lentils group, which is on top of what you've already been eating on Stage One. The exciting part about Stage Two is that the extra carb will give you even greater satiety while kicking your metabolism into even higher gear.

I recommend adding your additional carb during the day when being active allows you to burn it off for energy. At night, as our bodies wind down, we don't need carbohydrates for energy. That's why it's best to stick to lean protein and veggies later in the day.

Keep journaling. On Stage Two, writing down what you eat lets you know that you are doing the program correctly and you'll always know where you stand in terms of meeting your daily fiber goal.

CARBOHYDRATES PERMITTED ON STAGE TWO

Stage One Carbs:
- ☞ 1 serving of any cereal with 20–25 grams of carbohydrate and 12–13 grams of fiber per serving
- ☞ A minimum of 4 high-fiber crackers, containing at least 5 grams of fiber and no more than 2 grams net carbohydrate per serving
- ☞ 1 serving of fruit

Plus Stage Two Carbs (choose one of the following):
- ☞ 1 serving of fruit
- ☞ 1 serving of beans, peas, or lentils (refer to the Miracle Carb Bible for portion size and carb content)

SAMPLE STAGE TWO JOURNAL

DATE	CARB (A)	FIBER (B)
BREAKFAST		
Egg-white omelet with sautéed mushrooms and onions	0	4
¾ cup blueberries	15	5
4 high-fiber crackers	28	20
Coffee or tea	0	0
LUNCH		
Large chopped salad	0	6
4-ounces grilled chicken	0	0
F-Factor Vinaigrette	0	0
Unsweetened iced tea	0	0
SNACK		
Small apple	15	4
4 tablespoons PB2 (prepared)	0	0
1 tablespoon Polaner Sugar Free Raspberry Jam with Fiber	5	3
Water or zero-calorie flavored water	0	0
4 high-fiber crackers	28	20
DINNER		
Green salad with ginger dressing	0	3
1 cup miso soup	0	0
4-ounce sashimi	0	0
1 glass sake	5	0
DESSERT		
Fudgsicle Popsicle, no sugar added, fat-free	0	0
TOTAL	**96**	**65**

A – B = C

Total Carb	Total Fiber	Net Carb

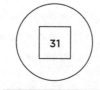

31

<45 g NET CARB

A

B

GET ENOUGH SLEEP

A healthful night's sleep—typically about 7.5 hours for adults—is important when you are trying to lose weight. What you may not know is that the amount and quality of sleep you get affects two hormones, leptin and ghrelin, that are factors in weight. Ghrelin is the hormone that stimulates appetite, while leptin's job is to signal the brain when you are full. When you are well rested, these hormones work in balance, and when you are not, they don't. Lack of sleep sends leptin levels plummeting, and when that happens, you don't feel satisfied after you eat. Lack of sleep causes ghrelin levels to rise, stimulating your appetite. If you sleep poorly, you may find yourself in a perfect storm for weight gain.

A study published in the journal *Sleep Medicine Reviews* found that when sleep was restricted to four hours per night over two nights, leptin (the hormone that tells our brain when we have eaten enough) dropped by 18 percent, while levels of ghrelin (the hormone that tells our brain when we are hungry) increased by an average of 28 percent. In other words, being sleep deprived at night can lead us to feel hungry during the day—even though we've had enough to eat.

THE SCOOP ON ARTIFICIAL SWEETENERS

I'm constantly asked about artificial sweeteners and here's the scoop: Nonnutritive sweeteners are a safe, healthy alternative to the sugar found in many of the foods and beverages we routinely consume. Simply by replacing sugar with a nonnutritive sweetener, you can cut your caloric intake significantly, resulting in weight loss. Saving 100 calories a day translates to about 10 pounds a year! However, switching to nonnutritive sweeteners does not give you free license to eat more. Nor will it break you of sugar cravings, because studies have found that whether it comes from sugar or a nonnutritive sweetener, sweetness itself drives desire for foods and drinks that taste sweet. So the bottom line is this: Nonnutritive sweeteners are helpful for weight loss, but use them sensibly and in moderation for foods that need sweetening.

FREQUENTLY ASKED QUESTIONS

On Stage Two, why do you recommend adding an extra fruit or serving from the beans, peas, and lentils group?

Having an extra serving provides greater satiety and it allows for more variety each day. The carbs you will be eating fill your glycogen tanks without causing them to overflow, so instead of burning glucose for energy the body gets it by burning fat.

Do I still need to have a snack in the afternoon?

Yes, an afternoon snack is mandatory. It only takes a few hours after you've had your lunch before your blood sugar starts to drop, giving you that late-day slump in energy and craving for a quick pick-me-up food. While most of us grew up hearing our mothers say, "Don't spoil your appetite for dinner," I say the opposite. Eating a snack that incorporates fiber and protein will always ensure that you won't sit down at the dinner table ravenous, leading you to overeat or inhale the bread basket.

What exercise do you recommend adding on Stage Two?

On Stage Two, I really urge you to add weight training to your fitness routine, because weight lifting adds muscle mass, which in turn increases metabolism and enables your body to burn more calories even when you are at rest. Research has shown that for every pound of muscle that you have added, you burn an extra 45 calories per day. By adding an extra 10 pounds of lean muscle mass, you can burn approximately 400–500 calories a day. That adds up to 1 pound of fat loss every week without doing anything else. For more on exercise, see Chapter 2: F the Gym.

STAGE THREE: THE HOMESTRETCH

Duration: Until you reach your goal weight

Focus: Add two servings of carbohydrate. Choose from any of the following:

☞ Starch: breads, cereals, and grains; starchy vegetables; crackers and snacks; beans, peas, and lentils

☞ Fruit

☞ Milk and yogurt

Total Net Carb: 65 grams per day

Total Fiber Goal: 35 grams per day or more

What to Expect: Lose approximately 1–2 pounds per week

During Stage Three, you will be adding two more servings of carbohydrate in addition to what you were eating on Stage Two. Your fiber goal remains 35 grams per day, and your goal for net carbohydrate is now 65 grams per day. You now have the freedom to choose which foods you would like to add to your diet. This is what allows you to customize the Miracle Carb Diet to your own likes and lifestyle. If you don't see your choices in the Miracle Carb Bible, just check your food's nutrition label and calculate the net carbohydrate per serving by subtracting the fiber content from the number indicated for total carbs.

You're almost there! Stage One introduced you to new ideas about eating and losing weight, and by now you've really changed your entire approach to eating and put yourself on a healthy new course. Stage Two gave you even more knowledge and confidence, and now you have a good understanding of how the foods you eat affect the way you feel and how you look. You're trusting yourself more to make the right choices, and your body is thriving.

On Stage Three, the physiological changes will become more apparent. No doubt your clothes have already become looser, but now you will begin to see very noticeable improvements in your overall health and continued weight loss. Exercise is becoming an enjoyable habit instead of a nuisance, and your muscles are getting toned. This is an exciting period of change for you. At this point, people are *really* starting to take notice, and you deserve to soak up all that positive energy. There's no better fuel than affirmation to keep you motivated as you head into the homestretch.

WHAT CARBS SHOULD I CHOOSE?

For optimal weight loss and to keep things simple for you, on Stages One and Two your food choices were limited. Now you are ready to make choices for yourself based on what works. It's important during this time to look closely at the Miracle Carb Bible and food labels. If you are like me, you like big portions. I want a lot of food with as few calories as possible. I want the most bang for my buck, and you should, too. On Stage Three, you'll learn that some foods have very small serving sizes because they are calorically dense. Take sushi rolls, for example. At first glance, you might think a sushi roll contains very little rice. However, the average sushi roll contains 1 cupful of rice, and if you were to look at the Miracle Carb Bible, you'd see that one serving of rice is equal to 3 slices of white bread. So while it is perfectly fine to have that sushi roll, just keep in mind that you will be using up all of your additional carbs for the day. There's nothing wrong with that. It's your choice. That's why it is so important to know how much of any food is equal to one serving of carbohydrate. When you know this, you can make wise decisions.

WHAT IS PB2?

Powdered peanut butter! How is that even possible?

A unique chemical-free process removes more than 85 percent of the fat from premium-quality peanuts. Essentially, the oil is squeezed out of roasted peanuts and what remains is this delicious powdered peanut butter—all natural with no artificial sweeteners or preservatives. Just mix PB2 with water to get the same consistency as full-fat peanut butter, with all the flavor and far less calories from fat. You can purchase PB2 online, and some health food stores stock it as well.

Comparison of Peanut Butter vs. PB2
2 tablespoons peanut butter = 200 calories, 16 grams fat
2 tablespoons PB2 = 45 calories, 1.5 grams fat

THE DIET: STAGE THREE

All the foods from Stages One and Two, plus two more servings of carbohydrates from any of the following:

☞ Starch: breads, cereals, and grains; starchy vegetables; crackers and snacks; beans, peas, and lentils
☞ Fruit
☞ Milk and yogurt

Total Net Carb: 65 grams per day

SAMPLE STAGE THREE JOURNAL

DATE	CARB (A)	FIBER (B)
BREAKFAST		
4 high-fiber crackers	28	20
2-ounce smoked salmon	0	0
2 tablespoons low-fat cream cheese	0	0
Tomatoes, onion, and capers	0	2
1 cup strawberries	15	4
Coffee or tea	0	0
LUNCH		
Steak Fajitas in high fiber tortilla with sautéed peppers and onions (recipe on page 285)	10	10
Unsweetened iced tea	0	0
SNACK		
F-Factor Cinnamon Apple Bar	27	12
1 cup nonfat cappuccino	15	0
DINNER		
Stir-fried shrimp with mixed vegetables (broccoli, carrots, celery, and bell peppers)	0	6
1/3 cup brown rice	15	2
DESSERT		
1/2 cup Arctic Zero Frozen Desserts	0	0
Decaffeinated coffee or tea	0	0
TOTAL	110	56

A – B = C

Total Carb	Total Fiber	Net Carb

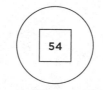

54

<65 g NET CARB

| A |

| B > 30 |

GRAB A BAR

No snack is quite as convenient as a bar, and F-Factor Bars are super high in fiber. They contain 27 grams of carbohydrate and 12 grams of fiber, so just one bar fulfills 50 percent of your recommended daily intake of fiber. They are more satisfying than a cookie and just as delicious in three tasty flavors: Fudge Brownie, Banana Walnut, and Cinnamon Apple.

STAGE THREE APPROVED FOODS

I highly recommend these products on Stage Three because now that you are given more variety, the supermarket aisle can seem a little overwhelming at first. These will help you narrow the field and get you familiar with great high-fiber choices.

CEREALS

Simply Fiber
- → Serving Size: ¾ cup
- → Calories: 100
- → Total Carbohydrate: 31 grams
- → Fiber: 14 grams
- → Net Carbohydrate: 16 grams

All-Bran Original
- → Serving Size: ½ cup
- → Calories: 80
- → Total Carbohydrate: 23 grams
- → Fiber: 10 grams
- → Net Carbohydrate: 13 grams

All-Bran Extra Fiber

→ Serving Size: ½ cup
→ Calories: 50
→ Total Carbohydrate: 20 grams
→ Fiber: 13 grams
→ Net Carbohydrate: 7 grams

All-Bran Bran Buds

→ Serving Size: ⅓ cup
→ Calories: 70
→ Total Carbohydrate: 24 grams
→ Fiber: 13 grams
→ Net Carbohydrate: 11 grams

Fiber One

→ Serving Size: ½ cup
→ Calories: 60
→ Total Carbohydrate: 25 grams
→ Fiber: 14 grams
→ Net Carbohydrate: 11 grams

Nutritious Living Hi-Lo (Original, Vanilla Almond, and Maple Pecan)

→ Serving Size: ½ cup
→ Calories: 90
→ Total Carbohydrate: 13 grams
→ Fiber: 6 grams
→ Net Carbohydrate: 7 grams

Nature's Pat Organic SmartBran

→ Serving Size: ½ cup
→ Calories: 80

- → Total Carbohydrate: 24 grams
- → Fiber: 13 grams
- → Net Carbohydrate: 11 grams

Arrowhead Mills Puffed Wheat

- → Serving Size: 1 cup
- → Calories: 60
- → Total Carbohydrate: 12 grams
- → Fiber: 2 grams
- → Net Carbohydrate: 10 grams

Kellogg's FiberPlus Antioxidants Cinnamon Oat Crunch

- → Serving Size: ¾ cup
- → Calories: 110
- → Total Carbohydrate: 26 grams
- → Fiber: 9 grams
- → Net Carbohydrate: 17 grams

BREAD

The Baker Flaxseed European Style Bread

- → Serving Size: 1 slice
- → Calories: 100
- → Total Carbohydrate: 18 grams
- → Fiber: 5 grams
- → Net Carbohydrate: 13 grams

Mestemacher Three-Grain Bread

- → Serving Size: 1 slice
- → Calories: 120
- → Total Carbohydrate: 24 grams

- → Fiber: 6 grams
- → Net Carbohydrate: 18 grams

Wonder Stoneground 100% Whole Wheat Bread
- → Serving Size: 1 slice
- → Calories: 90
- → Total Carbohydrate: 16 grams
- → Fiber: 2 grams
- → Net Carbohydrate: 14 grams

Arnold Sandwich Thins 100% Whole Wheat
- → Serving Size: 1 sandwich thin
- → Calories: 100
- → Total Carbohydrate: 22 grams
- → Fiber: 5 grams
- → Net Carbohydrate: 17 grams

Arnold Bakery Light 100% Whole Wheat
- → Serving Size: 1 slice
- → Calories: 40
- → Total Carbohydrate: 9 grams
- → Fiber: 2.5 grams
- → Net Carbohydrate: 6.5 grams

Thomas' 100% Whole Wheat Breakfast Thins
- → Serving Size: 1 breakfast thin
- → Calories: 100
- → Total Carbohydrate: 22 grams
- → Fiber: 5 grams
- → Net Carbohydrate: 17 grams

Thomas' 100% Whole Wheat Bagel Thins

- → Serving Size: 1 bagel thin
- → Calories: 110
- → Total Carbohydrate: 24 grams
- → Fiber: 5 grams
- → Net Carbohydrate: 19 grams

Thomas' Light Multi-Grain English Muffins

- → Serving Size: 1 muffin
- → Calories: 100
- → Total Carbohydrate: 26 grams
- → Fiber: 8 grams
- → Net Carbohydrate: 18 grams

Weight Watchers 100% Whole Wheat Bread

- → Serving Size: 2 slices
- → Calories: 80
- → Total Carbohydrate: 16 grams
- → Fiber: 6 grams
- → Net Carbohydrate: 10 grams

Flat Out Hungry Girl Foldit Flatbread 100% Whole Wheat with Flax

- → Serving Size: 1 flatbread
- → Calories: 90
- → Total Carbohydrate: 15 grams
- → Fiber: 7 grams
- → Net Carbohydrate: 8 grams

La Tortilla Factory 100% Fat Free Tortilla

- → Serving Size: 1 tortilla
- → Calories: 90

- → Total Carbohydrate: 24 grams
- → Fiber: 8 grams
- → Net Carbohydrate: 16 grams

La Tortilla Factory Smart & Delicious Low Carb, High Fiber Large Size Tortilla

- → Serving Size: 1 tortilla
- → Calories: 80
- → Total Carbohydrate: 18 grams
- → Fiber: 12 grams
- → Net Carbohydrate: 6 grams

CRACKERS AND SNACKS

High-Fiber Crackers

- → Serving Size: 1 cracker
- → Calories: 12
- → Total Carbohydrate: 7 grams
- → Fiber: 5 grams
- → Net Carbohydrate: 2 grams

Ruffles Light Original Fat Free Potato Chips

- → Serving Size: 1 ounce (15 chips)
- → Calories: 80
- → Total Carbohydrate: 17 grams
- → Fiber: 1 gram
- → Net Carbohydrate: 16 grams

Pringles Original Reduced Fat Potato Crisps

- → Serving Size: 1 ounce
- → Calories: 140

- → Total Carbohydrate: 17 grams
- → Fiber: 1 gram
- → Net Carbohydrate: 16 grams

Bare Fruit 100% Organic Baked-Dried Cinnamon Apple Chips

- → Serving Size: 12 grams
- → Calories: 29
- → Total Carbohydrate: 8 grams
- → Fiber: 1 gram
- → Net Carbohydrate: 7 grams

Glenny's Soy Crisps, Lightly Salted

- → Serving Size: 18 grams
- → Calories: 70
- → Total Carbohydrate: 9 grams
- → Fiber: 1.5 grams
- → Net Carbohydrate: 7.5 grams

Glenny's Soy Crisps, Creamy Ranch

- → Serving Size: 18 grams
- → Calories: 70
- → Total Carbohydrate: 9 grams
- → Fiber: 1.5 grams
- → Net Carbohydrate: 7.5 grams

Fiber Gourmet Lite Snack Crackers (Cheese, Nacho Cheese, Wheat)

- → Serving Size: 1 bag
- → Calories: 80
- → Total Carbohydrate: 20–22 grams
- → Fiber: 12 grams
- → Net Carbohydrate: 8–10 grams

Pop Secret 100 Calorie 94% Fat Free Mini Bag

→ Serving Size: 1 mini bag
→ Calories: 100
→ Total Carbohydrate: 23 grams
→ Fiber: 4 grams
→ Net Carbohydrate: 19 grams

Flat Out EdgeOn Baked Flatbread Four Cheese Crisps

→ Serving Size: 15 chips
→ Calories: 130
→ Total Carbohydrate: 15 grams
→ Fiber: 5 grams
→ Net Carbohydrate: 10 grams

Nabisco Wheat Thins Reduced Fat Snack Crackers

→ Serving Size: 16 crackers
→ Calories: 130
→ Total Carbohydrate: 22 grams
→ Fiber: 2 grams
→ Net Carbohydrate: 20 grams

Nabisco Triscuit Reduced Fat Crackers

→ Serving Size: 7 crackers
→ Calories: 120
→ Total Carbohydrate: 23 grams
→ Fiber: 3 grams
→ Net Carbohydrate: 20 grams

Ryvita Light Rye Crispbread

→ Serving Size: 2 slices
→ Calories: 80

- → Total Carbohydrate: 17 grams
- → Fiber: 3 grams
- → Net Carbohydrate: 14 grams

Shibolim Whole Wheat Sesame Crisp Snax

- → Serving Size: 9 Crisp Snax
- → Calories: 50
- → Total Carbohydrate: 11 grams
- → Fiber: 2 grams
- → Net Carbohydrate: 9 grams

Yehuda Matzos Whole Wheat Matzo

- → Serving Size: 1 matzo
- → Calories: 100
- → Total Carbohydrate: 23 grams
- → Fiber: 4 grams
- → Net Carbohydrate: 19 grams

Finn Crisp Multigrain Thin Crisps

- → Serving Size: 2 slices
- → Calories: 40
- → Total Carbohydrate: 10 grams
- → Fiber: 2 grams
- → Net Carbohydrate: 8 grams

Wasa Hearty Grain Crispbread

- → Serving Size: 1 slice
- → Calories: 45
- → Total Carbohydrate: 11 grams
- → Fiber: 2 grams
- → Net Carbohydrate: 9 grams

PASTAS

Fiber Gourmet Light Pasta (Penne and Rotini)
→ Serving Size: 2 ounces uncooked
→ Calories: 130
→ Total Carbohydrate: 42 grams
→ Fiber: 18 grams
→ Net Carbohydrate: 24 grams

Fiber Gourmet Light Mac-mmm-Cheese
→ Serving Size: 2.5 ounces uncooked
→ Calories: 160
→ Total Carbohydrate: 50 grams
→ Fiber: 18 grams
→ Net Carbohydrate: 32 grams

Barilla PLUS Penne Pasta
→ Serving Size: 2 ounces uncooked
→ Calories: 210
→ Total Carbohydrate: 38 grams
→ Fiber: 4 grams
→ Net Carbohydrate: 34 grams

Ronzoni Tri-Color Garden Delight Rotini
→ Serving Size: 2 ounces uncooked
→ Calories: 210
→ Total Carbohydrate: 42 grams
→ Fiber: 2 grams
→ Net Carbohydrate: 40 grams

Ronzoni Smart Taste Rotini

- → Serving Size: 2 ounces uncooked
- → Calories: 170
- → Total Carbohydrate: 40 grams
- → Fiber: 5 grams
- → Net Carbohydrate: 35 grams

De Cecco Whole Wheat Fusilli

- → Serving Size: 2 ounces uncooked
- → Calories: 180
- → Total Carbohydrate: 35 grams
- → Fiber: 7 grams
- → Net Carbohydrate: 28 grams

Bionaturae Organic Whole Wheat Fusilli

- → Serving Size: 2 ounces uncooked
- → Calories: 190
- → Total Carbohydrate: 42 grams
- → Fiber: 5 grams
- → Net Carbohydrate: 37 grams

Gia Russa Whole Wheat Roman Rigatoni

- → Serving Size: ¾ cup uncooked
- → Calories: 200
- → Total Carbohydrate: 40 grams
- → Fiber: 5 grams
- → Net Carbohydrate: 35 grams

Wild Harvest Organic Whole Wheat Penne

- → Serving Size: ¾ cup uncooked
- → Calories: 210

- → Total Carbohydrate: 41 grams
- → Fiber: 5 grams
- → Net Carbohydrate: 36 grams

DeBoles Organic Whole Wheat Angel Hair

- → Serving Size: 2 ounces uncooked
- → Calories: 210
- → Total Carbohydrate: 42 grams
- → Fiber: 5 grams
- → Net Carbohydrate: 37 grams

DESSERTS

F-Factor Bars (Banana Walnut, Cinnamon Apple, Fudge Brownie)

- → Serving Size: 1 bar
- → Calories: 150–160
- → Total Carbohydrate: 26–27 grams
- → Fiber: 12 grams
- → Net Carbohydrate: 14–15 grams

Swiss Miss Sensible Sweets Diet Cocoa (25 calories)

- → Serving Size: 1 packet
- → Calories: 25
- → Total Carbohydrate: 4 grams
- → Fiber: 1 gram
- → Net Carbohydrate: 3 grams

Sugar Free Jell-O Gelatin

- → Serving Size: 1 Jell-O
- → Calories: 10

- → Total Carbohydrate: 0 grams
- → Fiber: 0 grams
- → Net Carbohydrate: 0 grams

Reddi-wip Sugar Free, Fat Free Whipped Cream

- → Serving Size: 2 tablespoons
- → Calories: 5
- → Total Carbohydrate: 1 gram
- → Fiber: 0 grams
- → Net Carbohydrate: 1 gram

Tofutti Chocolate Fudge Treats

- → Serving Size: 1 bar
- → Calories: 30
- → Total Carbohydrate: 6 grams
- → Fiber: 0 grams
- → Net Carbohydrate: 6 grams

Fudgsicle No Sugar Added Pops

- → Serving Size: 1 pop
- → Calories: 40
- → Total Carbohydrate: 9.5 grams
- → Fiber: 2 grams
- → Net Carbohydrate: 7.5 grams

Creamsicles Sugar Free Pops

- → Serving Size: 2 pops
- → Calories: 40
- → Total Carbohydrate: 12 grams
- → Fiber: 3 grams
- → Net Carbohydrate: 9 grams

Arctic Zero Frozen Desserts

→ Serving Size: ½ cup
→ Calories: 37
→ Total Carbohydrate: 6 grams
→ Fiber: 2 grams
→ Net Carbohydrate: 4 grams

HealthSmart Chocolite Chocolate Caramel Pretzel Snack Bites

→ Serving Size: 2–3 pieces
→ Calories: 45–67.5
→ Total Carbohydrate: 11–16.5 grams
→ Fiber: 8–12 grams
→ Net Carbohydrate: 4 grams

HealthSmart Chocolite Protein Cookies N Cream Bar

→ Serving Size: 1 bar
→ Calories: 95
→ Total Carbohydrate: 17 grams
→ Fiber: 9 grams
→ Net Carbohydrate: 8 grams

HealthSmart Calcium Bites

→ Serving Size: 1 piece
→ Calories: 30
→ Total Carbohydrate: 8 grams
→ Fiber: 7 grams
→ Net Carbohydrate: 1 gram

Glenny's All Natural 100 Calorie Brownies

→ Serving Size: 1 brownie
→ Calories: 100

- → Total Carbohydrate: 12 grams
- → Fiber: 7 grams
- → Net Carbohydrate: 5 grams

Fiber Gourmet Lite Frosted Brownie/Lite Cinnamon Crumb Cake

- → Serving Size: 1 brownie/crumb cake
- → Calories: 90
- → Total Carbohydrate: 31 grams
- → Fiber: 12 grams
- → Net Carbohydrate: 19 grams

Fiber One 90 Calorie Chocolate Fudge Brownies

- → Serving Size: 1 brownie
- → Calories: 90
- → Total Carbohydrate: 18 grams
- → Fiber: 5 grams
- → Net Carbohydrate: 13 grams

Vitalicious Banana Nut VitaTops

- → Serving Size: 1 VitaTop
- → Calories: 100
- → Total Carbohydrate: 25 grams
- → Fiber: 9 grams
- → Net Carbohydrate: 16 grams

Kashi Oatmeal Dark Chocolate Soft-Baked Cookies

- → Serving Size: 1 cookie
- → Calories: 130
- → Total Carbohydrate: 20 grams
- → Fiber: 4 grams
- → Net Carbohydrate: 16 grams

Nabisco Newtons Blueberry Brown Sugar Fruit Thins

→ Serving Size: 3 thins
→ Calories: 140
→ Total Carbohydrate: 21 grams
→ Fiber: 2 grams
→ Net Carbohydrate: 19 grams

Nabisco 100% Whole Grain Fig Newtons Minis

→ Serving Size: 1 pack
→ Calories: 130
→ Total Carbohydrate: 26 grams
→ Fiber: 2 grams
→ Net Carbohydrate: 24 grams

Popsicle Sugar Free Orange, Cherry, Grape Pops

→ Serving Size: 1 pop
→ Calories: 15
→ Total Carbohydrate: 4 grams
→ Fiber: 0 grams
→ Net Carbohydrate: 4 grams

Tofutti Vanilla Cuties Sandwiches

→ Serving Size: 1 sandwich
→ Calories: 130
→ Total Carbohydrate: 17 grams
→ Fiber: 0 grams
→ Net Carbohydrate: 17 grams

Skinny Cow Vanilla Ice Cream Sandwiches

→ Serving Size: 1 sandwich
→ Calories: 150

- → Total Carbohydrate: 30 grams
- → Fiber: 3 grams
- → Net Carbohydrate: 27 grams

Skinny Cow Chocolate Truffle Bars

- → Serving Size: 1 bar
- → Calories: 100
- → Total Carbohydrate: 19 grams
- → Fiber: 3 grams
- → Net Carbohydrate: 16 grams

Skinny Cow Chocolate with Fudge Cones

- → Serving Size: 1 cone
- → Calories: 150
- → Total Carbohydrate: 29 grams
- → Fiber: 3 grams
- → Net Carbohydrate: 26 grams

Skinny Cow Fudge Bars

- → Serving Size: 1 bar
- → Calories: 100
- → Total Carbohydrate: 22 grams
- → Fiber: 4 grams
- → Net Carbohydrate: 18 grams

Skinny Cow Mint Ice Cream Sandwiches

- → Serving Size: 1 sandwich
- → Calories: 150
- → Total Carbohydrate: 30 grams
- → Fiber: 3 grams
- → Net Carbohydrate: 27 grams

Ciao Bella Blood Orange Sorbet Bars

- → Serving Size: 1 bar
- → Calories: 60
- → Total Carbohydrate: 16 grams
- → Fiber: 0 grams
- → Net Carbohydrate: 16 grams

Ciao Bella Mango Sorbet

- → Serving Size: ½ cup
- → Calories: 120
- → Total Carbohydrate: 30 grams
- → Fiber: 1 gram
- → Net Carbohydrate: 29 grams

FREQUENTLY ASKED QUESTIONS

I've made great progress, and I think I have the hang of this now. Why keep journaling?

I recommend you continue journaling for at least another two weeks. This will ensure that you are meeting your fiber goals and not exceeding your net carb quota for the day. But don't worry—you don't have to journal forever. After two weeks, I suggest you keep journaling for three days a week just to help keep you on track while you're eating a greater variety of carbohydrates.

How do I know if I am choosing the right foods on Stage Three?

I always recommend choosing whole foods first such as sweet potatoes, whole grains, and fruits. If you're opting for a processed food, be sure to refer back to the nutrition label and recommended Stage Three products.

How do I determine what a high-fiber carbohydrate is?

Carbohydrates that contain 5 grams of fiber or more are considered high fiber. Foods that contain less than 5 but at least 2 grams of fiber are good sources of fiber. Foods that contain less than 2 grams of fiber are considered low fiber. Remember that the more fiber a food contains, the more slowly it digests and affects your blood sugar levels. Plus, fiber keeps you feeling fuller longer on fewer calories and fewer net carbs.

Do I have to add all three servings of carbohydrate on Stage Three?

No, you don't have to add all three additional carbs every day. While it is important to remember that we are adding in more high-fiber carbohydrates to keep your metabolism boosted and for continued weight loss, you might find that some days you simply don't feel the need to eat all three servings. I myself find that on some days I am content to eat as if I were on Stage Two or even possibly Stage One.

Will I ever be able to have dessert? What about my birthday or anniversary? Salad isn't what I'd call a party, Tanya!

Of course you can have dessert. Yes, enjoy holidays and birthdays and the same for treats. On the Miracle Carb Diet there's no reason you should ever feel deprived. But let's agree on one point: Treats and fancy desserts are not meant to be daily indulgences. By definition they are to be enjoyed occasionally, which I find makes them all the more special anyway. And moderation is key, even when we are talking about eating birthday cake. Just take a small slice, or opt for a piece of dark chocolate or a bowl of berries with low-fat whipped cream instead. Take your time! Eat your treat slowly and savor it. Taste isn't the only sense to engage here. Appreciate the texture—the crunchiness or the smooth creaminess. Enjoy the aroma. Make sure each of those three bites is worth it. There's nothing worse than treating yourself to a dry, mediocre cake that ends up costing you 300 calories! I would much rather build the anticipation by thinking of my very favorite dessert, and then indulge in 300 calories' worth of the most delectable cake or éclair. Finally, if your friends are all ordering dessert and you spot fruit on the menu, this is the time to bend the rules by having a serving of fruit at night instead of during the day. Cheating doesn't have to be defeating!

Now that I can have bread, is it better for me to use olive oil or butter?

Normally I would opt for heart-healthy monounsaturated olive oil. However, when I do treat myself to a piece of bread, I prefer to use butter. Surprised? A teaspoon of olive oil and a teaspoon of butter *both* have 45 calories and 5 grams of fat, so nutritionally, they're the same. However, we tend to use only a teaspoon or pat of butter at a time. Since butter is a solid form, we have a visual cue about how much we are using. Olive oil is a liquid and it's harder to know how much of it soaks into our bread each time we dip it. So I recommend you go with butter.

What should I do if I had a bad eating day?

It is important to remember that weight loss is not a sprint—it's a marathon. If you trip and stumble, just get up, dust yourself off, and keep moving toward your goal. The one thing you never want to do is skip your next meal to compensate. Skipping meals slows down your metabolism and can make you ravenous when you do decide to eat again. Don't punish yourself; rather than starving, get back on track at your very next meal and focus on eating healthfully for the rest of the day. At the end of the day, weight loss is determined by calories in vs. calories out. If you overindulged, clean up the rest of the day or hit the gym a little harder at your next sweat session to burn off those extra calories.

Do you recommend any supplements?

I recommend taking a calcium supplement with vitamin D. While some studies have shown that insoluble fiber, such as wheat bran, can leach calcium from bones because fiber binds with excess estrogen in the body (which has been tied to osteoporosis), there are also studies that show a diet high in fiber does the opposite, making these studies inconclusive. The F-Factor way has always been focused on health and longevity, so calcium-rich foods such as low-fat mozzarella, cottage cheese, yogurt, and fortified cereals are all included from day one, but we always recommend taking a calcium supplement. This is especially important for women. I suggest using Citracal Plus Bone Density Builder or any other Citracal product. The recommended amounts for calcium are 1,000 milligrams for men and women ages 19–50 and 1,200 milligrams for men and women ages 51 and up. Eating foods high in calcium is also advised, and you can find rich sources of both calcium and fiber in fruits and veggies such as berries, spinach, broccoli, and salad greens. Almonds are a good source of both nutrients, too.

STAGE FOUR: YOUR NEW NORMAL

Duration: For the rest of your life
Focus: You have reached your goal and now have the tools to maintain your goal weight within a 5-pound range
Total Net Carb: 65 grams per day
Total Fiber Goal: 35 grams per day or more

Congratulations, you have reached your goal weight! Welcome to the new you! Everything has changed—the way you think about food, how you live your life, how you perceive yourself, and even the way you are perceived by others.

Stage Four really isn't a stage as much as it is your new healthy state of being that will enable you to eat very well and maintain your weight loss for the rest of your life. You will continue eating as you did during Stage Three, so the real purpose of this maintenance phase is for you to reinforce those healthy choices, attitudes, and behaviors that are now your new normal.

Throughout this book, I've said the F-Factor way is a lifestyle approach to weight control, and by now you understand why. My clients are able to maintain their weight loss, many for the first time, because F-Factor's principles are simple to embrace no matter who you are and how you live. Plus, the Miracle Carb Diet itself is all about enjoying foods that you love every day—delicious meals, satisfying snacks, desserts, and spirits, too. If you are a home cook, you'll be proud to serve up F-Factor recipes. And if you frequently dine out, entertain, or travel, you know that great F-Factor choices abound wherever you go.

Your diet—now defined as the foods you choose to eat—is as good as it gets. Not only do you select wisely from all the food groups, but you are also meeting or even exceeding the Academy of Nutrition and Dietetics's recommended daily intake of fiber. In these pages, you've learned about the many benefits of fiber—satiety, detoxing, anti-aging, increased metabolism, stable blood sugar, and more—and you are already realizing them all. You know this because you can see and feel the difference.

Best of all, you have the knowledge and tools to sustain your success, and that is the golden ticket when it comes to living a longer, stronger, healthier, and more satisfying life. Your weight is no longer a nagging problem; now you feel free to eat and drink what you like, you have energy to spare, you feel more in control, and you have a brighter outlook, too. Bravo!

SUSTAINING SUCCESS

The F-Factor is not a diet per se, because it's really a model for healthy living and weight management. The term *diet* is derived from the Latin word *diaeta*, which means daily routine—hence our diet comprises the kinds of foods we habitually eat. Nowhere in this definition does it say anything about a rigid eating regimen that's not forgiving of slipups. I developed F-Factor with a keen appreciation for life's twists and turns and our need to be adaptable when things don't go according to plan. In other words, I never want you to fear what you eat. If you overeat at Thanksgiving, so be it. If you have a second cocktail each evening while on vacation, don't sweat it. Of course you want to be diligent day in and day out, but minor setbacks won't take you out of the game.

Keep your eyes on the big picture: Eating and exercising the F-Factor way will give you the body you want, more energy, and a real zest for living. You can count on it!

Everyone starts Stage Four feeling a bit apprehensive. It's like going from student pilot to flying your first solo flight. Here are some of my favorite tips to keep you confident and in control as you settle into maintaining a healthy weight and lifestyle:

New Clothes, New You

Many of my clients ask what they should do with clothes that no longer fit. In the back of their minds, I know what they are thinking: *Shouldn't I keep a few dresses and trousers just in case?* No! Declare your weight and clothes sizes and stick to them. If you suddenly feel your skirt is getting snug or your suit jacket puckers across the shoulders, go back to journaling. The secret to lasting weight loss is to know what works and keep doing it. So please don't pack away your old clothes. Have them tailored or give them away to someone who needs them.

Shut the Door on Foods and Habits That Made You Fat

Now that you understand how eating refined carbs promotes weight gain, you know why eating the right carbs will enable you to reach your goal weight and maintain it without struggle. Sure, there will be times when you want to treat yourself, and you can on the Miracle Carb Diet. But to resist the draw of foods that led you to gain weight, I say put them behind you for good. Ban them from your pantry if you can and do your best to ignore them when you are grocery shopping, at the mall or movie theater, or dining out. Cutting refined carbs out of your diet will bring an end to cravings, but be forewarned that going back to those foods puts you in the danger zone.

FREQUENTLY ASKED QUESTIONS

What do I do at a wedding or long event?

Always plan ahead! Assume there won't be a morsel of food served at whatever wedding or event you're going to. Eat a large snack beforehand, so you arrive at the reception with a full stomach. It's much easier to eat and drink sensibly when you aren't hungry. Always scan the hors d'oeuvres scene to see what's available so you don't wind up grabbing at whatever happens by on a waiter's tray. I also tell my clients to order a beverage, alcoholic or not, first thing to keep their hands busy. A great trick for women is to carry a clutch bag in one hand and a drink in the other. That way you'll eat less, mingle more, and spare yourself 600–800 empty calories along the way—and that's before you even sit down to dinner.

I have a busy schedule, which makes it difficult for me to spend a lot of time cooking complicated healthy meals. Any ideas about throwing together fast and healthy options?

This book includes more than one hundred recipes, all of which are super simple, require few ingredients, and are packed with flavor. Go Greek one day, Indian or Asian the next. Variety will keep your diet interesting. The best part is if you don't like to cook, you don't have to. From day one you can easily dine out for breakfast, lunch, snacks, cocktails, and dinner!

Make sure to keep well stocked with healthy options. Tried every recipe in the book? Not to worry: Go to FFactor.com for great recipe ideas! And healthy, tasty recipes are available by the thousands on various cooking and food sites across the web. You could prepare a new dish that's F-Factor-friendly every single day for a year and still not run out of options. Be adventurous!

What do I do if I overindulge on vacation or at a party, or just fall off the wagon?

I'll say it again: Losing weight is not a sprint. It's a marathon, and you are setting the pace for the rest of your life here. But life is short, and you should be enjoying yourself on holidays and vacations. Indeed you can, by following what I call the 90–10 Rule. Commit to eating well 90 percent of the time and the remaining 10 percent allow yourself wiggle room for indulgences. Just do the math: There are 365 days a year, so that 10 percent leeway translates into 36.5 days when you can kick back and coast a bit. Everyone deserves a slice of cake on their birthday! I never want to see someone sidelined by their diet when they could be out celebrating. I'm not giving you carte blanche to go wild most Saturdays, of course, because you need to be thoughtful about when, how, and how often you indulge. Any treat worth having is one you'll enjoy to the max!

2

F THE GYM

Diet trumps exercise when it comes to weight loss, plain and simple. If you're overeating, all the exercise in the world isn't going to make you lose pounds. On the flip side, dieting alone isn't going to give you the body you want, because unless you develop lean muscle, your weight loss will leave you looking skinny and flabby. Finding the right combination of the two is what will give you the best physique you've ever had. I call it "skinny-strong."

There is plenty of evidence suggesting the kind of physical activity associated with gym rats and reality-show boot camps does not melt away the excess pounds. Why is that? It still comes down to hunger and overeating. While exercise burns calories, which you must do to lose weight, it also makes you hungrier. Many people follow their workout with a well-intended snack or sports drink that's packed with calories, not realizing that they just negated what they burned off exercising. One poor choice made in an impulsive minute can easily undo the fifty laps you just swam or the five miles you just jogged. That's why you need to make proper diet the foundation of your weight-loss program and support it with the best types of physical activity.

Lots of people make the mistake of thinking that any exercise is exercise, and it's all the same. There are two types of exercise—cardio and strength training—but few realize how differently these impact the body. People come to me all the time after they've spent endless hours walking, running, or spinning without losing the weight they desire. In some cases, they even gain despite a rigorous cardio regimen. Why? Consider for a moment that 1 pound of fat is equivalent to about 3,500 calories. In order to lose 1 pound of fat in a week, you would need to either cut out or burn 500 calories every day. The problem is you would have to run an hour a day for a week just to burn that 1 pound. The good news is that you can achieve that same 500-calorie deficit simply by switching out your morning bagel for a bowl of high-fiber cereal with fresh berries. Effortless!

On the Miracle Carb Diet, eating fiber-rich carbohydrates in combination with lean protein creates the caloric deficit you need to shed weight without hunger. That's part one of the two-part weight-loss equation. Building strength through exercise is the other critical component. Adding muscle through weight training will not only give you the toned look you want, but building muscle mass will actually boost your metabolism as well.

MUSCLE: THE OTHER MIRACLE

Who wants to be skinny and flabby after all their hard work dieting? Why put in all this effort if you're not going to look good naked or in a bathing suit? For many Americans who are sedentary, excess calories are stored as fat. What your body can't immediately use, it stocks away as a precaution. Diet alone can't completely outsmart that natural process. You need some muscle to win this fight for you.

I've had male clients who are physically strong, but their muscles are buried beneath what I call a "fat sweater." They may work out regularly, but their diet is so full of refined carbs that it produces a layer of fat that hides their six-pack abs. I also have female clients who devote hours to aerobic exercise yet never see much of a change in their weight and shape.

If you're losing weight solely by cutting calories, as much as 25 percent of what you lose could be muscle, according to some studies. That's why starvation diets don't work for long; they actually slow down the metabolism, making it harder to lose weight and easier to regain weight. Lost muscle means lost space in the larger of your two storage tanks for glucose, and that, in turn, means excess glucose heads straight to your fat cells for storage.

Our bodies constantly burn calories, even when we're doing nothing. This resting metabolic rate is much higher in people with more muscle because muscle is more metabolically active than fat; the more muscle you can add from weight training, the higher your metabolism will be. Muscle is our calorie-burning machine, and maintaining lean muscle mass means we can eat more without gaining weight.

On the Miracle Carb Diet, pairing fiber and protein at every meal and snack fires up your metabolism even more. That fiber-protein combination is useful for another reason, too: Protein contains essential amino acids that the body needs to build lean muscle. If you are actively lifting weights, it's even more important to give your system the protein it needs to repair, maintain, and build new muscle tissue. Building lean muscle and eating lean protein go hand in hand. That's why on the Miracle Carb Diet, you'll eat ample amounts of protein throughout the day, always with fiber. It's easy to do with an ultra high-fiber cracker, along with any of the protein toppers you'll find on Stage One of the diet.

The simplest and most effective way to build lean muscle is through strength training by lifting weights or doing resistance exercises. Mind you, strength training won't necessarily drive down the numbers on the scale, since muscle weighs more than fat, but you have to remember that muscle is what gives you a lean, toned look. Another big plus: A pound of muscle burns about 35–50 calories per day. That means that by adding 10 pounds of muscle to your frame, you can burn 350–500 more calories per day, which is like burning off about a pound of fat every seven to ten days.

People often focus too much on the number they see on the scale. In my office, in addition to using the scale, I measure a client's percentage of body fat, because that's the more important gauge for body leanness. Someone who weighs 110 pounds with 30 percent body fat is probably what I would describe as "skinny-flabby"—not overweight, but not at all lean, either. And definitely not the "lean-toned" look we're striving for. If you have a lot of muscle, you'll naturally weigh more on the scale. A person may weigh 180 pounds, but if only 10 percent of it is fat tissue, then he probably has well-developed muscle. I recommend buying an inexpensive body fat monitor to track your body fat composition, or if you go to a gym, simply do it there.

LEAN FOR LIFE WITH FOOD AND FITNESS

Have you seen pictures of Jack LaLanne as a senior citizen? The fitness pioneer was lean and strong enough to perform fingertip push-ups without breaking a sweat at an age when many people struggle to make it up a single flight of stairs; he was buff well into his nineties, and he didn't get that way doing Zumba. He did it through a combination of sound nutrition and weight training.

Muscle loss is a natural part of the aging process, and it is why we tend to gain weight as we get older. We lose an average of 5 percent of our muscle mass every ten years after the age of thirty-five. Let's assume you don't do any weight training: By some estimates, you would need to cut as many as 450 calories per day for each decade just to maintain your current weight. Few Americans plan to eat less with each passing birthday—the rate of adult obesity attests to it. But you can defy nature and avoid the excess birthday baggage with regular strengthening exercise, which rebuilds muscle. Eating the F-Factor way further enhances the benefits.

Maintaining muscle mass is extremely important from an anti-aging standpoint. Men and women begin to lose lean muscle tissue starting in their forties, and the process accelerates once we hit our fifties. Menopause causes a decline in the female hormone estrogen, which can spell higher cholesterol, a loss of bone density, and a greater propensity for gaining weight. For menopausal women who are inactive, this is a good time to start exercising—with particular emphasis on weight training.

Only a basic and progressive strength-training program can effectively slow down the rate of muscle loss. A deficit in muscle mass means you're burning fewer calories each day, which is why people tend to gain weight year after year even if they watch what they eat. Another issue that comes

Exercising increases the level of endorphins in your brain. Endorphins have a chemical structure similar to morphine; raising endorphin levels can increase your feeling of well-being. Studies have shown that regular strength training can have a marked positive effect on those who are chronically depressed. A Duke University study found that forty-five minutes of exercise three times a week, including strength training, was as effective against depression as taking an antidepressant.

with aging is declining bone health; one out of two women over the age of fifty is diagnosed with osteoporosis. Proper nutrition along with a regimen of weight-bearing exercise is your best ally for good bone health.

GETTING STARTED WITH WEIGHT TRAINING

Women often worry that they'll bulk up from weight training, but I can tell you that the right routine will give you the svelte look you want. You don't need to join a gym or invest in expensive equipment. Good athletic shoes and a few pairs of dumbbells will do just fine. The best way to become lean is to challenge yourself by lifting more weight in fewer repetitions. The benefit of lifting more weight is that it engages and develops all of your core muscles, which won't happen if you are doing many repetitions lifting light weights. Concentrate on building muscle mass for weight control and you'll benefit more than if you'd gone out for a forty-minute run.

I caution you not to overthink exercise. It's easy to feel like an outsider if you are walking into a fancy gym for the first time in years. Why go that route if you don't want to? Buying simple weights to use at home is cheap and easy. Dress for comfort, not fashion, although I bet you'll want to treat yourself to a shopping spree once you start seeing some results!

A sensible weight-training program should work all the major muscle groups: chest, back, arms, shoulders, and legs. Work out for about thirty to forty minutes, three days a week if you can, but even two days of weight training each week will make a difference. Be sure to let the muscles rest between workouts—about forty-eight hours between sessions.

Begin by lifting hand weights or doing resistance exercises. For best results, and to make the most of your time and effort, you should lift enough weight to feel sufficiently challenged. Your muscles should feel heavy after 8–12 repetitions—so fatigued you really can't do more. As you get stronger, it's important to increase your weight load by about 5–10 percent—again to the point of fatigue after 12 reps. You can invest in resistance bands for at-home training, but basic push-ups are also very effective. Try one to three sets of 8–12 repetitions (if you can do more than that, kick it up a notch to something harder).

Morning workouts will rev your metabolism for the rest of the day. Performing short bursts of exercise for ten to fifteen minutes every few hours helps, too.

While one of the attractions to weight lifting is the fact that it can be done conveniently and inexpensively at home, I recommend scheduling some sessions with a qualified fitness trainer who can assess your readiness and show you how to best use weights to meet your goals. Learning proper form and technique will help you get into weight lifting safely, and the right routine will get the results you want. If you can't afford a trainer, consider buying a DVD or online program by a well-regarded fitness expert. Online trainers are also a hot new trend and especially good if you have self-motivation but want an expert to turn to for advice and new workout routines as you build stamina and flexibility. Just keeping a weekly exercise log may also provide the accountability you need to keep up the good work.

Some people see exercise as an opportunity to socialize, while for others it's a precious chance for some alone time. Rule of thumb: Do what makes you happy and you're more likely to stick with it. Know that exercise is going to build more than physical fitness for you; it's going to boost your self-confidence along with your metabolism, and when you start to feel good about yourself, you are going to feel a stronger commitment to taking care of yourself. Positive outlook and positive outcome become self-perpetuating.

Once you achieve your goal weight on the Miracle Carb Diet, you are going to be able to eat more food without gaining back body fat. It doesn't get better than that! You will have sped up your metabolism and added enough muscle mass to be one of those people you've always envied—the lean and healthy ones who seem to go through life eating whatever they want without guilt or fear of becoming fat. Now you have what you need to make exercise an enjoyable part of your lifestyle. So get going already! I promise it will add years to your life and life to your years.

EXERCISE PREP SHEET

☞ **Always check with your doctor first.** If you're overweight and have other clinical conditions, such as high blood pressure, muscle or joint problems, cardiovascular health concerns, or diabetes, check with your physician before starting a strength-training regimen. You need to take those into consideration and proceed smartly.

☞ **Set short-term goals.** That's one of the biggest psychological pluses of weight training vs. cardio: Twenty minutes with some 2-pound or 5-pound weights is far less daunting than the prospect of an hour-long run. But don't expect miracles overnight. Lasting results require a lasting effort.

☞ **Keep a journal.** Record your progress. Share your achievements with supportive family members and friends. Feed your ego instead of your belly—boast a little!

☞ **Choose activities you'll enjoy, and switch it up if you get bored.** If you don't like the smell of chlorine, then swimming laps is going to feel like punishment. Similarly, find a weight-training routine that keeps you interested and motivated. Boredom and frustration are among the biggest reasons why people quit too soon when they first start an exercise program.

☞ **Set aside a regular time.** Planning ahead will keep you on track and limit the excuses.

BENEFITS OF WEIGHT TRAINING

Boosts Metabolism: You burn more calories, even while at rest.

Regulates Appetite: Vigorous exercise increases body temperature, which has been shown to suppress appetite.

Strengthens: Even moderate weight training can increase a woman's strength by 30 to 50 percent. Strength training builds stronger muscles as well as stronger connective tissues and better joint stability. You will stand taller and your core will feel firmer.

Slims: Muscle takes up less space than fat; lean muscle gives your body a toned, slender appearance.

Increases Bone Density: Weight training has been shown to increase spinal bone mineral density. This, coupled with dietary calcium, helps reduce the risk of osteoporosis.

Improves Heart Health: Studies have shown that weight training can help lower LDL ("bad") cholesterol, increase HDL ("good") cholesterol, and lower blood pressure.

Lowers Risk for Diabetes: Research suggests that weight training may improve the way the body processes sugar, which in turn may reduce the risk of diabetes.

Enhances Mood: In a Harvard study, strength training during a ten-week period reduced clinical depression symptoms more successfully than standard counseling.

Anti-Aging: Research shows that the average woman who strength trains two to three times a week for two months swaps 3.5 pounds of body fat for nearly 2 pounds of muscle; on average, for every pound of muscle you gain, you burn 35–50 more calories a day.

3

A TALE OF
THREE DIETERS

"It was the best of times, it was the worst of times . . ." The famous line from Charles Dickens's classic *A Tale of Two Cities* could easily describe the conflicted relationship most dieters have with food. It sustains us, it delights us, it torments us, and, sadly, it sometimes controls us. In my practice, I see such a cross-section of people—from teenagers to grandparents, from soccer moms to celebrities—all of them landing in my office with the same desperate plea: "Help me lose this weight once and for all!" Although the circumstances of their lives are always unique, as dieters, the situations they find themselves in are not. There is a commonality to the challenges they face, the obstacles they overcome, and the triumphs they achieve. Sharing some of their stories, I hope, will empower and motivate you as you work toward your goal to be fit for life, the F-Factor way.

LAURA

When I met Laura, she was a busy thirty-nine-year-old mother of three who gave up her career on Wall Street to raise a family. She had just begun working part-time again as a consultant now that her youngest son was in school.

"It's hard to remember a time when I *wasn't* trying to lose some weight," Laura admitted at her first appointment. "I was never supermodel skinny, but I guess my weight really became an issue when I went away to college and for the next four years gained and lost and regained the classic freshman fifteen plus some. One of the reasons I look so happy in all my graduation pictures is because the gown hid the fact that my final semester was a four-month binge!" I smiled in spite of myself. Laura's self-deprecating sense of humor was a classic defense mechanism; I knew it was a way to deflect the disappointment she felt. She would rather disparage herself than imagine others silently doing so. I've seen many Lauras (and her male counterparts) over the years: They're the ones who've always been the pleasantly "pudgy" girl or guy, and they compensate for it by being the funny one or by assuming some Wonder Woman or Superman role, such as confidant or protector. Lauras are so preoccupied seeking acceptance from others that they ignore their own needs and potential.

After college, Laura told me, she slimmed down on a demanding fad diet, but as she entered the working world, adhering to it got tougher and tougher, especially once she was entertaining clients, many of whom were men who favored porterhouse steaks with loaded baked potatoes and a slab of cheesecake afterward. Tailored suits and killer heels diverted attention away from Laura's waist and hips. She dressed beautifully, but secretly she yearned to be a couple of sizes smaller.

Fifteen years and three babies later, Laura still had those skinny clothes hanging in the back of her closet, but now they were more than a few sizes too small. It wasn't as if she had just let herself go and hadn't been trying to get back into shape all this time: Laura was always the first in her circle of girlfriends to try whatever hot new diet was on the market. "I'd always lose at first, then it would stop working or I couldn't stick to it, and I'd end up regaining it all," she recounted. Her mother had even urged her to try Weight Watchers, but there was something too old-fashioned about it to Laura. "Just not my style," she concluded. Joining some program where prepackaged assembly-line diet meals would arrive on her doorstep seemed equally bleak.

When she fell in love and got engaged, Laura drove her fiancé crazy by changing their wedding date so she'd have more time to lose weight. A drastic juice diet got her down to the size 4 gown she wore on her wedding day, "but I can't believe how pale and sickly I actually looked when I watch the videos now," Laura said. "I felt so weak and tired. I found out later that I was anemic." When she had her first baby, Laura shot up to 160 pounds during her pregnancy. "First I craved pasta, and I could eat a mound of linguine in a single sitting," she remembered. "Then I went on a four-month frozen yogurt spree—thinking it was health food!"

"Rookie mistake," I informed her with a smile. "Guess what? Each has about 240 calories, so actually they're about the same."

Laura's pregnancy weight never fully came off. She would drop 10 or 20 pounds every six months or so on her diet of the moment, then boomerang back. "I got skinny the wrong way so many times," she lamented. By the time she came to me, she was nearing her heaviest weight ever—and the prospect of losing 35 pounds seemed monumental.

Reentering the working world had Laura motivated—for now. The yo-yo cycle is one of the toughest to break. But the Miracle Carb Diet is actually ideal for people like Laura, since they don't have to give up any favorite foods, and there's no reason for them to get bored. The variety of fiber-rich foods is huge and growing by the day. On the Miracle Carb Diet, Laura would be adding things to her daily menu, not just omitting them. Eating more would also rev up her metabolism, so she wouldn't hit the plateaus that routinely happen on a radical deprivation diet that confuses your body into producing more fat.

"I'm not going to lie to you," I cautioned Laura. "You're going to have to want this, and you're going to have to work for it. It's not absolutely effortless, and I can't do it for you, or I would. But you *can* have the body you want. You are the one in the driver's seat; I'm in the passenger seat. I can give you directions and help you navigate bumps in the road. I'll cheer you on along the way, but I don't control your outcome. Only you do. You're going to reach your destination because you decided to drive the entire way yourself."

We talked for a while about the biggest pitfalls Laura had encountered on previous diets, and together, we were able to identify some of her biggest risk factors:

Fatigue. Laura was constantly catering to her family's needs, whether it was running everyday errands, playing the corporate wife role for her successful husband at gala fund-raisers, or volunteering to help out at every school and extracurricular activity her kids were involved in. On top of that, Laura's widowed father was in poor health, and Laura was an only child. Excited as she had been to go back to work twenty hours a week before her father's illness, Laura was now feeling guilty about the job, much as she enjoyed it. On the nights when the family wasn't eating takeout or grabbing dinner on the run at a drive-thru, Laura didn't even sit down to make herself a plate, opting instead to graze off her kids' plates. "Or I'd just skip dinner altogether to make up for something fattening I had at lunchtime or the baked goodies someone brought to the office," she said.

Depression. Laura had lost her mother to emphysema several years earlier, and even though she was keeping up a cheerful façade for her family's sake, the prospect of losing her father, too, was hitting her hard. When she was alone at home or waiting at the hospital while her dad underwent tests or treatments, Laura often sought comfort in food. "I don't know why," Laura told me, "because I'd always just end up feeling worse."

"That's because food can't solve your problems—or push them to the backburner," I explained to her. "Eating for all the wrong reasons will only leave you exasperated. So the next time you find yourself heading for a binge, instead of giving in to weakness, do the things that will make you physically and emotionally stronger. Eat really well, which means keeping to your normal schedule of meals and snacks and choosing healthy foods you enjoy."

Laura lost 6 pounds in her first week on the Miracle Carb Diet and was elated. She told me getting started on Stage One was easy because she knew exactly what to eat. "I just did the plan and, best of all, I wasn't walking around tired and hungry." When Laura came to see me two weeks later, she not only looked thinner, but she was looking noticeably healthier as well. "I'm getting my energy back," she explained. "I'm sleeping much better at night, and now I start the day refreshed and ready to go." I was happy that Laura was trying different Miracle Carb recipes, too; it turns out her kids loved my Hearty Bolognese as much as my three do (see recipe on page 158). Laura had even scoped out several gyms around town and had found one with the kind of friendly, low-key vibe she was hoping for. I was thrilled. "You're doing everything exactly right," I praised her.

By the seventh week, however, Laura arrived for her appointment looking exasperated and announced that she had hit a wall. After losing 20 pounds in steady increments, the scale suddenly showed nearly a 10-pound gain. I could tell by the look on Laura's face that she felt defeated.

"Don't worry," I assured her. "Remember that you have to go into this with a goal of being good 90 percent of the time. No one is perfect, and no one expects you to be 100 percent all the time. You had a bad patch, but the good news is that you caught yourself before falling down. Just go back on Stage One for a week or two and I know you'll be fine." Laura smiled as she welled up with tears.

"Laura, what's going on?" I gently probed.

"Maybe I'm just not meant to be one of the skinny girls," she said. "I should just accept myself the way I am. What's it really matter whether my jeans are a 12 or a 4? At the rate I'm going, I'll be forty before I reach my goal weight."

"Well," I pointed out, "the months until then are going to pass quickly and you're going to turn forty whether you're thin or not. Close your eyes for a minute and visualize yourself celebrating your fortieth in the most perfect way you can imagine. What does that look like? Where are you? Describe it to me."

Laura took a deep breath and sighed. "At a beautiful tropical resort with my husband. Our room overlooks lush gardens, and you can smell the flowers from the balcony. There's a beach with a private little cove where we take a bottle of Champagne to toast the sunset. It's romantic and just incredibly peaceful."

"What are you wearing?"

"A white bikini with a sheer, sexy sarong that flutters in the breeze when I walk."

"So you're relaxed and happy with yourself. That's good. Are you at all uncomfortable with your weight while you're on this dream vacation?" I asked.

"Not at all," Laura said.

"Okay, open your eyes," I told her. "You can still have that, you know. Do you still want it?"

"Yes, of course I do," she replied readily.

"This is yours for the taking," I said.

I urged Laura to go back and reread her food journal to see if she could pinpoint what had made her falter or to see if there was a pattern that led up to her making some poor choices. She called me a few days later to report back.

"I think it was a combination of a couple of things," she said. "First, I was feeling really good about myself and all the compliments I was starting to get. My husband was so supportive and proud of me; he even took me out for a special dinner to celebrate when I reached my twenty-pound mark. He thought I deserved a treat, and I guess I went overboard that night—ordering fried calamari as an appetizer and lobster ravioli for my entrée. Then we split this incredible tiramisu for dessert. It was downhill from there. I felt like I'd blown it that week already, so why bother, it wasn't going to matter that much more if I had a slice of pizza for lunch or some buttered popcorn when we went to the movies that weekend. At the same time, though, my dad was making the decision to enter hospice care, and I just didn't want to face what that meant. It's still really hard on me. He hasn't been eating much, and I started making lots of fattening comfort foods to try to get his weight up a little. And, of course, I ended up eating right along with Dad. I don't know. I'm really stuck now and don't see a way out of this anytime soon," she concluded.

"I'm really sorry about your father," I began. "I know that's a tough situation to cope with, but you've made a really important connection between that pain and your way of seeking comfort in food. Going forward, that kind of self-awareness is really going to help you recognize and defuse such emotional tripwires. Next time, what if instead of eating you make plans to meet a friend for coffee or just talk on the phone, right after visiting your dad? And keep using your journal, too. It's not just for listing food—it's also a tool to help you understand your emotional eating patterns."

There was one last thing I needed to address with her, and it was a delicate subject.

"You need to keep your well-meaning husband from sabotaging your efforts to lose weight," I said. "While you absolutely can still dine out on this diet, taking you out for a heavy dinner when you are struggling was counterproductive. Let him know how much you value his support and suggest other ways to show it, like a gift certificate for a spa day, or surprising you with flowers or jewelry or tickets to a show or concert you've always wanted to see. And when the time feels right, you might want to ask how he feels deep down about you getting thin. Sometimes spouses feel threatened by their partners becoming attractive to other people."

Laura put herself back on Stage One of the diet and immediately started losing again. She also joined the gym, where she began lifting weights and attending a salsa cardio class that helped clear her head and lift her mood. Regaining a sense of control over her own body gave her confidence she needed to better cope with the crisis she couldn't control—her father's illness. Laura and her husband started working on their relationship, too, and Laura reached her goal weight shortly after her fortieth birthday. She celebrated with three delectable bites of tiramisu, and her husband surprised her with tickets for a Caribbean vacation.

Last I heard, Laura had her eye on a chic white bikini.

JEFF

Jeff, a smart, successful businessman in his forties, had worked hard to get way ahead of the pack. He earned his success every single day, and I knew he had the drive to get in shape if he could just approach his health the same way and make losing weight a goal to check off his life's task list. If you met him at a party, Jeff would strike you as comfortably mature and confident—not the type who tries to cling desperately to youth, but not exactly willing to let it go without some fight, either. Jeff's thriving family, beautiful home, and prized Maserati were all testament to his strong work ethic. This wasn't a man used to giving up.

I could tell right away that Jeff was one of those achievers who seemed to be successful at everything he set his mind to—except dieting. The guy could crunch numbers like Warren Buffett when it came to analyzing a corporate budget, but keeping a spreadsheet on his spreading middle was something he steadfastly avoided. Over the years, Jeff had gradually gained weight—the result of eating and drinking well—and often.

But Jeff knew that self-indulgence would exact a terrible toll down the road, and he was starting to worry about his state of health. Several of Jeff's friends had already suffered heart attacks or undergone coronary bypasses, and his business partner, who was obese, was being treated for type 2 diabetes. Jeff's father died at sixty-four from colon cancer, and Jeff worried about his increased risk of developing the disease. At Jeff's last physical exam, his doctor voiced concern about high blood pressure and cholesterol and put Jeff on Lipitor. Results of Jeff's stress test put him slightly below average—more reason for concern. Both Jeff's doctor and wife had been pushing him to lose weight, and his wife had convinced him to seek my help after she saw me talking about the F-Factor philosophy on a morning talk show.

"I need some sort of plan here. Being fit always used to just come naturally to me. I played sports all through high school and college, and working out was a big part of my life," Jeff recalled. "Now I don't have time to even get in an occasional game of squash or a good bike ride—forget regular trips to the gym. I'd give anything to have back the body I had in my twenties, but that ship has sailed, I know."

"Why do you think that?" I asked. I'm always curious when I hear people saying it's "too late" to have the body they want. The right combination of diet and exercise can give even someone in his or her seventies a sculpted physique. I have plenty of clients who look and feel far better after forty than they did at twenty. Jeff looked at me as if I were crazy.

"My metabolism has slowed down with age," he said. "My body doesn't burn it off the way it used to."

"You're right," I told him. "After age forty your body starts to lose muscle mass and when that happens your metabolism slows," I explained. "The good news is you can reverse that by making some time for strength training. A basic routine with hand weights and resistance exercises will do the trick, and it's something you can do at home without a trainer. Exercise and the Miracle Carb Diet equal success, so the onus is on you to do both.

"Let me ask you something," I continued. "When you were climbing the corporate ladder, how did you go about becoming as successful as you are?"

Jeff brightened. "I pinpointed what company I wanted to work for, then did my homework and found out what it would take to get hired there. And once I was in the door, I set my sights on the executive suite and the biggest corner office in the place. I don't know how else to explain it: I knew what I wanted and I just went for it. I took every class and seminar I could to build my résumé, and I worked seventy-hour weeks. When the other junior execs were out drinking at the sports bar on Friday night, I was still in the office busting my ass. If there was a big project in the works, I made sure I was part of the team. I didn't want to end up one of those guys who's resigned to spending his entire life in the middle. It's not like I was some wunderkind or visionary genius. I wanted to be at the top, and I basically didn't stop until I got there."

"So," I said, "once you got where you wanted to be, you were able to just kick back and enjoy the view from that corner office, right?" Now Jeff looked at me like I was *really* crazy.

"Are you kidding?!" he asked. "I have to work just as hard—harder, even—to hold on to it."

"What I'm hearing in all this is that when you make something a priority, it's going to happen," I summed up. Jeff nodded slowly in agreement. I could tell it was starting to click into place for him.

"It's time to make yourself the priority," I announced. "There is no plan B here. Plan B is for losers—no pun intended. It's plan A or bust."

Here's a funny thing I've learned in this business: Men are like soldiers with diets. Women like to accessorize, but men appreciate a smart strategy and a logical plan of action. You spell out what needs to be done, and they tend to do it. Men sometimes trip themselves up when they become overconfident about their weight loss. They start to tinker with the rules, so to speak, and the pounds start piling on again. Some guys knuckle down and start again—and some don't.

Jeff followed Stage One with a diligence that didn't surprise me in the least, losing 8 pounds in two weeks. But then he missed two appointments and disappeared. He sent an apologetic e-mail: His firm had thrown itself into a heated competition to acquire a major international client, and Jeff's already demanding schedule went into overdrive. He was traveling constantly and getting little sleep between the jet lag and long hours spent in meetings. Most evenings he was either hosting lavish business dinners at hot restaurants or ordering in and eating alone in his hotel suite. Evenings alone were rough on Jeff. He missed his family, and a combination of loneliness and boredom usually drove him to raid the minibar in his room for overpriced, fattening snacks. Burning off some of the extra calories was hard when he was sedentary all day long. "Sometimes I can squeeze in a half hour in a hotel gym," he reported, "but that's rare." When he did manage a workout, he added, it was usually followed by a power breakfast with his business associates. He had stopped keeping his food journal because "I knew I was blowing it," but he gave me a rough idea of what was going on:

A big power breakfast meant a Western omelet, hash browns, orange juice, and coffee. Meetings through lunchtime, with a big deli spread set up for everyone. More coffee, with a tray of fruit, muffins, and cookies to munch on in the afternoon. Then he would take a quick break back in his hotel room to answer e-mails, call his family, and shower before meeting everyone again for predinner cocktails. He would usually raid the minibar for a can of nuts or a protein bar to hold him over until dinner. Down at the bar, Jeff would usually have a martini and whatever hors d'oeuvres the table had ordered—crackers and pub cheese, Buffalo wings, chicken satay. Then it would be dinner at a fancy restaurant, where Jeff would order a small green salad and prime rib with potatoes, or maybe a whole branzino with rice pilaf, wine, and dessert with a cappuccino. There would usually be a nightcap before heading back to the hotel suite. If he had a flight to catch, Jeff typically grabbed an Italian sub with chips at the airport.

Stress and being on the road were obviously taking a toll, causing Jeff to make poor choices. I immediately sent him the Miracle Carb list of what to eat in an airport, along with samples of Miracle Carb–friendly choices found on the menus of popular restaurants. Even if he wasn't eating in one of those particular chains, any restaurant would have menu options built around the same ingredients. Jeff also needed a reminder about portion control: The amount of food restaurants put on your plate is usually twice the normal portion the average woman should eat, and a man should only be eating three-quarters of what's on his plate.

"Always start with veggies and let their fiber start to fill you up so you're not relying so heavily on protein and starches to satiate your hunger," I reminded Jeff. I urged him to order first at the bar or restaurant to have more influence over choices, such as which appetizers to choose or whether to have dessert. Groups almost always go along with the first person to make a suggestion, and the waiter will likely look to you first to answer for the table, too, when asking if he should bring more bread or the dessert cart.

"Good health and a trim physique are the body's equivalent of the prime corner office," I said. "You want it, you deserve it, and you know you can have it."

Jeff corrected course by jumping back to the F-Factor way of doing things and even used his innate leadership skills to improve a challenging situation: "I just announced one afternoon that I was going to skip the cocktail hour and get in a workout before dinner, and two other guys immediately said it was a great idea and decided to join me. Within a few days, that had become the new routine for most of our group. I was able to sleep better at night right away, and I had more energy during the day."

"Just be on guard that you don't start rewarding yourself for the workout by overeating at dinner," I cautioned. "And keep yourself hydrated. Coffee and Diet Cokes aren't going to do that for you—you need to be drinking lots of water."

Jeff did end up with the trim, muscular body he had had in his youth and was able to lower his cholesterol and go off Lipitor. His wife even followed along on the plan with him and shed 9 pounds she had been trying to keep off without success, and both of them have been on maintenance for three years now. The international expansion of Jeff's company didn't doom him to an expanded waistline, and now that he's traveling overseas on a regular basis, Jeff has learned how to easily adapt the Miracle Carb Diet to the foreign cuisines he's enjoying.

"My variance is five pounds up or down," he says. "I've learned how to better eyeball portions. I know that the lid of a Starbucks cup is the equivalent of a serving of rice and that I can satisfy my sweet tooth with two cups of blueberries instead of a small handful of jelly beans.

"I love eating," he adds. "I like feeling full. The F-Factor approach and the specific Miracle Carb meal plans have taught me how to eat, not how to diet. Now that I've lost the excess weight and flab, I can tell that clients are taking me more seriously. They definitely see me as more disciplined, more focused."

When he treated his family to a ten-day Caribbean cruise over Christmas break, Jeff worried that the sprawling shipboard buffets, elegant dinners, and 24/7 snacking options would be too hard to resist, and he might end up slipping back into destructive old habits.

"You've waited a long time to take this vacation with your family," I reminded him. "You've all sacrificed a lot these past few years as you built up your career. This is about having a chance to really appreciate and enjoy their company and spend time with them, not about turning every meal into some three-ring circus.

"You're a skilled strategist," I said. "That's how you got where you are today. Just apply those same talents to taking care of yourself. Think of it this way: Before you go on this trip, you're going to look at your itinerary, check the weather, and pack only what you need so you're not lugging around suitcases full of stuff you don't need, right?

"And you're no doubt going to do a little research on your ports of call, to figure out in advance what you'd like to see and what activities you want to do.

"Approach eating the same way. Have a plan. Tell yourself before you go to dinner, 'I'm going to have that grilled tuna and a big salad tonight.' Order off the menu instead of doing the buffet. Eat a healthy snack in the afternoon so you aren't famished in the evening. There'll be a gym on board, so take advantage of it and keep up your workout routine. Take your wife dancing, learn how to windsurf—vacations are a great time to rev up your level of activity and have fun doing it."

Jeff came back from his trip tanned, trim, and triumphant. "It was a blast," he said. "Sure, I fell off the wagon—you couldn't expect me to ignore the buffet table completely—but I made sure that even that was planned and not impulsive. When I found myself tempted by all the food, I promised myself a cheat day. I ate whatever I wanted that day, felt like a bloated pig all night, and that was that. It was good to know that I can afford to make a bad choice now and then and fall right back into my F-Factor routine without missing another beat. This is how I eat now, and I feel good doing it.

"I know that I don't ever wanna go back!"

SOPHIA

I see many anxious twenty-seven- and twenty-eight-year-olds in my practice, and they're often motivated—initially, at least—by the same looming milestone: Their ten-year high-school reunions. Everyone has felt the pressure surrounding that kind of event, whether you're reconnecting with former classmates, an old flame, or distant relatives. You just want to present the very best version of yourself possible. Sophia was excited about returning to her small midwestern hometown as the polished career woman she had become, and she was determined to show up at her ten-year reunion looking nothing less than fabulous.

"I was the funny, fat girl in high school," she told me. "I had lots of friends, but not many dates. I went away to college and lost a lot of weight when a friend got me hooked on rowing. I loved it, and I never looked better. Then I moved to the city and got on the career track, and the pounds have been sort of sneaking back on over the past few years." None of her new friends was into rowing, so that had fallen by the wayside, and Sophia was eating most of her meals—if you could call them that—out. "Most of the time, I'm just going out for drinks after work with everybody, and whatever the bar's serving during happy hour becomes dinner," she said. On weekends, there always seemed to be a wedding or other event to go to, and Sophia would fill up on rich party food. "Everybody seems to be doing dessert parties for their showers now," Sophia said. "You can't leave one of those without feeling like you've just gained five pounds!"

"Sure you can," I interjected. "They didn't invite you because you're an

Olympic-class eater. They invited you because you're good company. Trust me, no one is going to gossip at work the next day about you only eating one mini éclair instead of five."

Sophia's party-like-it's-1999 lifestyle also meant she was waking up most mornings feeling hungover or sluggish from her overindulgences the night before; she rarely wanted anything but a cup of coffee for breakfast.

"I know, I know—it's the most important meal of the day," she said. "But I eat lunch fairly early and make up for it."

Lunch was usually a turkey panini or chicken salad sandwich from the Panera next door to her office. "Those are lean proteins. That's healthy, right?" Sophia asked.

"See for yourself," I said, pulling the restaurant's website up on my computer screen. I clicked on the menu and nutrition calculator.

"Here's your turkey panini," I showed Sophia. "It's showing up as 710 calories with 26 grams of fat and 68 grams of carbohydrate. There's 5 grams of fiber, so you can subtract that from the carb total, but you're still loading up on 63 grams of carb. Remember, one serving is 15 grams. And check out the protein—between the turkey and the cheese, you've got 53 grams of protein, or about 7.5 ounces. The average protein intake on the Miracle Carb Diet is 9 to 17 ounces a day. You multiply that by seven to convert it to grams, so figure 63 to 119 grams of protein daily." The secret to the Miracle Carb's fat-burning success is in combining your lean proteins with fiber at every meal.

Sophia's favorite chicken salad was "only" 690 calories but even worse on the carb count—90 grams, minus 5 grams from fiber. This time, Sophia did the quick math herself. "That's practically six servings of carbohydrates," she noted.

"Right," I agreed. "So would you sit down and eat six slices of white bread in one sitting? Of course not. But you've just done the equivalent of that. And that's before we even count the bag of chips that comes with each sandwich."

I scrolled through the deli's menu. "Here's a better option," I suggested. "This half chicken-apple salad has only 280 calories and a total of 15 carbs once you subtract the fiber. And it's got just under 17 grams of protein."

Sophia looked relieved. "So I can still go out on this diet? I was afraid you were going to tell me I had to pack hard-boiled egg whites and celery sticks in a brown bag to eat at my desk every day. That would be so pathetic."

I shook my head. "You are not going to starve or become a hermit. You're going to be eating *more* on the Miracle Carb Diet, not less. And you can go out as often as you like. We're changing how you eat, not how you live."

Sophia happened to be tall and pear-shaped. The extra weight had settled on her hips and thighs, and finding clothes with a flattering fit could be frustrating for her. "I spend a fortune on tailoring," she admitted. She had her eye on a knockout designer cocktail dress for her reunion and would need to lose 20 pounds to reach her goal weight. The reunion was in three months.

Needless to say, Sophia was highly motivated to lose the weight, but she made the mistake of thinking that she would lose even more quickly if she skipped snacks and ate less than the diet's daily food plan allows.

"It just seemed like a lot, and I knew I could tough it out and get by on less," she explained meekly when her steady weight loss suddenly slowed down drastically.

"There is plenty of food on this plan," I agreed, "but it's nutritionally balanced, and your actual intake is less than 1,400 calories per day. Your body needs to be properly nourished, and when you cut back too much, it goes into survival mode because it thinks it needs to hoard energy by storing it as fat."

Returning to the plan, Sophia was able to go to her reunion in the sexy cocktail dress she had been coveting, and she basked in the attention of old classmates who didn't even recognize their onetime fat friend.

Back in the city, though, Sophia let all the compliments she was getting lure her into complacency. "I had reached my goal. I was skinny and I thought that gave me license to eat whatever I wanted again," she later admitted. "That's what I had always envied about skinny girls. I assumed they could eat anything and not gain weight, and now I had joined that club."

At work, she helped herself to a Hershey's Kiss whenever she passed by the big glass bowl on the receptionist's desk and told herself it would be rude to refuse a slice of cake at the birthday, retirement, and promotion parties that cropped up every week in her big firm. When she went out with friends in the evening, she stopped choosing for herself and just went along with whatever decision the group was making about appetizers or another round of margaritas. On dates, Sophia worried about coming across as "finicky" or "high-maintenance," so she was reluctant to ask the waiter to take away the bread basket or serve her salad dressing on the side. If she was spending the evening home alone in front of the TV, she snacked on a bag of microwave popcorn or pretzels, or sometimes a late-night bowl of cereal with skim milk. In the morning, she was back to her old habit of rushing out the door without breakfast.

Sure enough, all those small lapses in judgment began catching up with her, and Sophia was doomed to learn the hard way that it doesn't take nearly as long to gain 10 pounds as it does to lose it. When she dragged herself guiltily back to my office, I knew it was time for tough love. Sophia was young, but she was at a critical turning point here: If she fell into a cycle of losing and regaining now, she could end up a lifelong yo-yo dieter. I knew she would be able to drop the weight she had regained so far; my bigger concern was whether she would make use of the maintenance tools the F-Factor gives every dieter. For lasting weight loss, it's important to stick with the framework of the diet that you know works. Eating fiber and protein at every meal is the cornerstone of the Miracle Carb Diet because it nourishes and satisfies hunger. Continuing with strength training boosts your metabolism. Exercise and the Miracle Carb Diet in combination is the key to taking weight off and keeping it off. Sophia had stopped keeping a journal—a mistake when you're on maintenance. Without a journal to review, it was hard to pinpoint exactly where things had gotten off track.

"You're giving in to three of the biggest psychological reasons why people overeat," I explained. "Boredom, for starters. Start writing things down in your food journal again, and see how often you're just eating something because it's there, not because you're hungry. The Hershey Kisses, the handful of nuts when you're out drinking, the cakes and other goodies being passed around at the office—that's all mindless eating. Okay?

"Now here's trap number two: peer pressure. Not being assertive about what you want or don't want to eat when you're out on a date or with a group of friends is a lame excuse to overeat. Most of that perceived pressure is all in your own mind, anyway. It's how you imagine people perceive you, not how they actually experience you. C'mon, do you honestly believe someone isn't going to ask you out again because you wanted salad dressing on the side or didn't share an appetizer? Would you *want* to go out with some creep who did? You're not five years old and vying for membership in the clean-plate club. You're a grown woman who wants to take the best possible care of herself. Look at you! You're beautiful! You buy the nicest clothes you can afford, and you'd rather buy one perfect Chanel lipstick than half a dozen cheap ones. You put the time and effort into your image, and you have reason to take pride in that. F-Factor taught you how to apply the same high standard to what you put inside your body. Eating well is an art, not a sport. F-Factor is your paint-by-numbers kit."

The third psychological reason behind Sophia's eating genuinely surprised her.

"You're tired," I said. "You're partying with your friends, you're not exercising, and you're starting the day with empty fuel tanks by skipping breakfast. You're cheating yourself out of the extra energy that fiber creates for you. When you're tired, you lose focus. You're not paying attention to things that become rote habit to you when you're following the F-Factor plan. Like portion control. You eat that bag of microwave popcorn without checking the nutrition label first and discovering that a bag is two servings, not one. You think you're being good when you order the poached salmon in a restaurant, but you don't eat only half and save the rest for lunch or dinner the next day. Even healthy foods like grilled fish come in unhealthy portion sizes in most restaurants."

Sophia renewed her commitment to herself and made another one a year later, when she married a wonderful guy who never even noticed the bread basket was missing from the table.

TOP MISTAKES DIETERS MAKE

1. **Skipping Breakfast:** Mom was right. It is the most important meal of the day, and going without food first thing in the morning puts your body into survival mode for fear it won't have fuel to burn for energy. Metabolism slows to compensate, and then your body starts storing calories you consume later in the day as fat. It just makes sense that we should eat based on our body's need for energy, which is why I always say eat breakfast like a king, lunch like a prince, and dinner like a pauper.

2. **Not Drinking Enough Water:** Dehydration mimics the symptoms of hunger, so you may be snacking when all you really needed was a glass of water. If the idea of sipping plain water seems pretty dull, make it more enticing by adding slices of fresh lemon, lime, orange, ginger, or cucumber.

3. **Overeating after Exercise:** Let your reward for working out be a flat tummy, toned legs, and buff arms, not a deep-dish pizza for lunch.

4. **Skipping Snacks:** Becoming overly hungry sets you up to overeat at your next meal. You can easily manage hunger by eating a healthy and filling snack, such as a piece of whole fruit, some high-fiber crackers, a wedge of Laughing Cow Light cheese, or a small handful of pistachios or almonds.

5. **Not Getting Enough Sleep:** Being sleep deprived affects hormones in a way that tell the brain that we're hungry even if we've just eaten.

4

THE FORK IS
IN YOUR HAND

We've all been there: It's holiday time and you merrily dig into your mother's buffet . . . and pack some up for later; for you relaxing at home Saturday night means TV and tearing open a fresh bag of chips and a nice tub of onion dip; it's time for your annual review at work and suddenly your chocolate cravings are off the charts.

Many of us have deep emotional ties with food and eating. Certain foods may take us back to happy times or offer us refuge from anger, sadness, or fear. People who struggle with their weight often have a tangled relationship with food; those who eat in response to emotional needs often find themselves caught in a vicious cycle of bingeing and self-loathing. The problem is food-induced bliss sometimes lasts only a few minutes; you come out of it feeling queasy, exhausted, and fearful of the new weight you'll gain. Understanding the feelings and situations that may lead us to overeat gives us the power to stop misusing food to cope. Many of the hours I spend coaching my clients revolve around this troubling food-emotion dynamic, teaching people how to break the cycle by really checking in with themselves and identifying feelings and issues that have absolutely nothing to do with being hungry. All of us, whether or not we struggle with our weight, expect what we eat to leave us satisfied. For those who use food to satisfy emotional needs, eating can be like feeding a bottomless pit. It doesn't have to be this way.

First, let's agree that being overweight can deeply influence how we feel and how we live. To show you what I mean, I'll use what I call my pitcher-and-dye demonstration. It goes like this:

Imagine I have an empty glass pitcher on my desk. I begin to fill it one cup of water at a time, and each of those cups represents a facet of your life. Let's say the first cup is your wonderful family. The next one is your health, and the cup after that is your career, and another marks your friends and community. The last cup of water may be your favorite hobby or pastime. The pitcher is now full, and it reminds you of how lucky you are to have such as full life. Now I take an eyedropper with red dye that represents your weight. I squeeze one drop, and immediately our water starts turning cloudy. Soon, all the water in the pitcher has a pinkish tint. I use this demonstration to make the point that being overweight affects much more than your appearance. Those extra pounds caused by an unhealthy diet can rob you of energy you'd draw on to really enjoy your family and friends. When you don't feel or look your best, are you as sexy as you want to be in the bedroom or as confident as you need to be in the board-room?

Flip open any magazine, turn on any television talk show, or browse the self-help aisle of any bookstore, and when the topic is dieting, I guarantee you that the terms *emotional eating*, *eating your emotions*, or some other variation of that theme will always come up. But believe me when I say that the reason one in three adults are overweight is not because they are sad, frustrated, or bored.

Emotions don't make you overeat.

As human beings, we have both rational thought and emotion. Are you overweight because of how you're feeling? Don't thin people feel angry, too? A pizza tastes delicious—no argument from me there—but it definitely won't save your marriage, jump-start your career, or give you a hug on a tough day.

The only problem eating solves is hunger, which is purely a biological need. You might think I'm heartless or harsh, like I'm blaming the victim who put on weight because they're going through an emotional time. Rest assured I am filled with empathy for anyone who struggles with their weight, but put your trust in my objectivity because it is based on everything I know about the science of nutrition and healthy weight loss.

I remember when Susan, a favorite client of mine, disappeared for a few weeks, then sheepishly reappeared in my office one morning. "You wouldn't believe what I've been going through," she explained as she got off the scale 8 pounds heavier than the last time I'd seen her. Her mother's dementia had worsened, and she needed to move her parents into assisted living; her daughter was getting married in a few months, and planning the big event already had Susan on her last frazzled nerve. On top of all that, her husband's company was laying off senior staffers, and he could be losing his job soon. Listening to her litany of very real, very scary crises, I knew that Susan was stretched to her limit taking care of everyone else, and she had relegated her own needs to the bottom of her to-do list. I truly ached for her as she poured out her heart and fought back tears.

"I'm so discouraged," she said. "I'm furious with myself for not having more self-control."

"I can see these issues just piling on you," I told her. "And if I thought for one second that eating would solve any one of these problems, Susan, I swear I would personally take you out for a deluxe hamburger and a large side of fries."

The fact that Susan was actually coping with so much stress was proof that she could manage her weight. "You've accomplished much more difficult things already," I reminded her. "You *can* control what you put in your mouth."

This was a terrible time, to be sure, yet it presented an opportunity for change, too. With F-Factor, Susan already had all the tools to help herself—she just needed to be reminded they were there and learn how to use them. We worked together to refocus and get back on a healthy food track. Taking control of what she ate and making good choices actually restored a sense of stability to Susan's life. A simple strength-training routine twice a week not only lifted her mood but also gave her the ego boost she needed by seeing the return of her toned arms, which had always been a point of pride for her. I had seen a similar response from many other clients as well. When you're feeling shattered, making yourself a priority by eating well and taking good care of your body is the best way you can start to put all the pieces back together. After all, being in a state of good health contributes to our overall sense of well-being. Our rational self knows that devouring a quart of ice cream won't fix our problems. Our emotional self can deny reason in favor of quick gratification. Stuffing yourself with comfort foods or going on a chocolate binge may release endorphins in your brain and give you a fleeting sense of well-being, but those endorphins are going to vanish just as quickly and surely as that pint of rocky road did, and you could end up feeling worse than you did in the first place.

I'm not going to give you some drill sergeant lecture here. I chose my line of work because what I wanted more than anything else in the world was to take care of people and to make sure everyone was as happy and well as they could possibly be. Please don't think for an instant that I'm discounting anyone's feelings, because I promise that nothing could be further from the truth. But setting you up for success means we have to rid your mind as well as your body of toxins, and I am determined to banish the victim mentality when it comes to losing weight.

I want you to start this diet not by looking in the mirror and saying you can't stand yourself, but by looking in the mirror and saying you respect yourself and want and expect the best for yourself. I know you may not like the way you look or the way you feel. I get it. No one wants to stay home from a wedding or party because they can't find anything flattering to wear. That's a crummy feeling. But you are changing that now; you will look and feel better in a mere matter of days on the F-Factor plan. The fact is good nutrition is incredibly powerful, and it starts working right away, beginning inside and moving to the outside. You've made that commitment to yourself, and you should congratulate yourself for that decision. The secret of success is having the courage to begin in the first place.

WHAT TYPE OF EMOTIONAL EATER ARE YOU?

Knowing what type of an emotional eater you are, and the feelings that make you want to eat, will help you diffuse and dismantle your emotional triggers. A large part of my coaching focuses on helping clients achieve greater self-awareness. It's hard to control what you do not understand. In my years of private practice, I've found that emotional eaters can be distinguished by type.

Idle Eater

Around food, you simply zone out, and eating has become a mindless habit for you. At work, you usually have a stack of cookies or a small pile of cheesy crackers on your desk from the supply you keep on hand in your snack drawer. You nibble away without thinking. Every time you pass by the reception area, you scoop up some jelly beans from the big bowl set out for clients. In the lunchroom, you always help yourself to the zucchini bread someone brought in to share or a cluster of grapes off the deli platter left over from advertising's big meeting. Idle eating isn't just a workplace phenomenon; it is just as prevalent among people who travel, who work by themselves, and who stay at home. You're automatically eating, whether it is because you are sitting in an airport or finishing whatever is left on your child's plate.

The Dark Cloud

Negative emotions rule the day for you. You're reeling from another argument with your spouse, child, or boss. You feel frustrated and defeated. Once the anger subsides, depression moves in. Why doesn't anyone understand what you're going through, how hard you're trying, how unfairly you're being treated? You know you'll feel better once you just calm down, and you can count on food to comfort you without ever asking how your day was or complaining about your foul mood. Fudge brownies are never judgmental.

Lonely Heart

Everyone feels lonely now and then, no matter how big a family or circle of friends they may have. But maybe you're having a tough time steering out of that skid right now: You just broke up with your boyfriend or girlfriend, or you're a single parent whose baby went off to college last week, or you moved to a different city to start a new job and you don't know a soul. Sometimes when it gets to you, you feed the void by ordering a pizza with extra cheese. What's that? It comes with a side of Buffalo wings and a liter of soda? It's like the universe is sending you a hug.

The Happy Camper

Life, from your perspective, shouldn't just be lived—it should be celebrated! And what better way to celebrate than with food? You happily gorge yourself at weddings and bar mitzvahs. You make those little pigs in a blanket everyone loves when the book club meets at your house. You congratulate yourself for going to the gym in the morning by rewarding yourself with a Starbucks Venti Mocha Frappuccino in the afternoon. When the gang at work meets that killer deadline on an important project, it's you who immediately volunteers to do the cupcake run. You're a holiday person, and you love going all out to make them special for everyone; those family feasts conjure up some of your warmest memories. Yeah, you know you really should lose some weight, but every time you start the latest fad diet, you're invited to someone's baby shower or birthday bash, or your husband wants to throw a big Super Bowl party, which you have to admit does sound like a lot of fun. Your philosophy is that life is short, and if you don't seize the day, you could miss out on something really good—like the pretzels at the Munich airport. When your boss treats you to dinner, why not have a second chocolatini and dessert?

The Peer Pressure Cooker

You hate conflict or confrontation, and you're just not hardwired to stand up for yourself. When friends sabotage your diet by ordering nachos for the table, or your mother-in-law insists you "at least try" her famous pecan pie and proceeds to cut you a huge slice, who are you to say no? At business dinners, you feel it's poor manners not to mirror the courses—and calories—your clients order. Besides, it's embarrassing to call attention to the fact that you're on some special diet. You wish you didn't have to worry about all this and could just eat like all your friends.

Chances are you identify with one (or maybe more) of these groups. Don't worry—you have lots of company. But you've decided it's time to make a change. By the time you finish reading this book, you'll be marching to the beat of your own drummer—and feeling great about it.

Look, no one is perfect, and no one needs to be. But that's no reason to settle for less than we can hope to be. No one strives for mediocrity, and I believe wholeheartedly that we are rewarded when we work toward being our best. Change may not happen overnight, but we can make it happen a little more each day. To give you an example, I struggle with the high expectations I hold for myself. I can be very self-critical when something is not going according to plan. Instead of becoming frustrated, now I hit the pause button and take a deep breath, collect my thoughts, and either adjust my goal or re-strategize.

It's the same approach I recommend for weight control, because there are so many obstacles that can complicate our best efforts. Food is cheap, plentiful, and readily available. Portion sizes tend to be ridiculously huge. Advertisers and the media entice us with images and messages equating food with happiness. Even the local supermarket feels like a miles-long gauntlet of temptation. (That's intentional, by the way: Ever notice how necessities like milk are all the way in the back? That's so you have to walk down a long aisle of cookies or chips or other non-staples to get there, increasing the chances of an impulse buy.)

To stay on course and overcome everyday obstacles, it's best to remove our emotional self from the driver's seat and let intellect take the wheel instead. Keep your eyes on the finish line—looking and feeling the way you want, being a good example for your children, and staying healthy.

Learning how to stop and check in with yourself throughout the day is an effective way to heighten your self-awareness. It's much easier to prevent a stumble in the first place than it is to stop a long, hard fall as it's happening. You have to become your own interrogator: Play around with different questions you can ask yourself to fend off the impulse to overeat. Here are a few that have proven effective with my most successful clients:

What purpose is this food serving for you?

Why are you eating if you are not hungry?

Will it fix the problem?

How are you going to feel about eating it three hours after you've finished?

Say you're feeling anxious about an important presentation you have to make for a big client your company is hoping to land, and you can't sleep. You've gotten up and wandered into the kitchen, where you're about to pour a big glass of milk to go with the chocolate cupcake you snatched from the batch your daughter is taking to the cheer squad's bake sale tomorrow.

Think about it: Does this cupcake provide anything your body needs to run properly?

Nothing. It just tastes good and helps me forget about the presentation for a while.

Will it fix the problem?

Won't change a thing... except maybe upset my daughter if she takes inventory of her cupcakes in the morning.

How are you going to feel about eating it three hours from now?

Guilty. Disappointed with myself.

Still not convinced? Then run through the drill a second time, substituting *losing weight* for *the food you're considering.*

What purpose will losing weight serve for you?

It will make me look better, feel better, and probably live longer.

Will it fix the problem?

Well, I would probably project a lot more confidence if I felt attractive, and the client will take me more seriously—I've seen all those articles about the negative stereotypes of overweight people in the workplace.

WAYS TO CONTROL EMOTIONAL EATING

→ Since hunger can trigger cravings, eat satisfying meals and snacks and stick to regular eating patterns.

→ Turn a blind eye (and nose) to tempting foods that you know are off-limits. Ban them from your home, desk, car, and handbag.

→ Satisfy the essence of a craving with something sensible. Tortilla chips are crunchy and salty, but deep-frying loads them with fat. Get the same taste sensation with whole grain pita bread, cut into wedges, lightly sprayed with cooking spray, sprinkled with salt or dried herbs, and toasted crispy brown.

→ Preempt a binge by doing what you can to avoid unnecessary stress, fatigue, and boredom. Also, sidestep rather than act on a craving. Call the old college roommate you've been meaning to catch up with. You're more likely to find a true friend on the phone than in the refrigerator. Try chatting instead of cheating. Or give yourself a sense of accomplishment by tackling some small chore, like finally cleaning out that kitchen junk drawer that gets jammed whenever you try to open it.

→ Visualize yourself as the in-control kind of person who you want to be.

→ Don't be ruled by your emotions. Deal directly with problems and feelings. There's no such thing as eating anger. Express it like a grown-up. If you're overwhelmed, sit down with your partner or a trusted friend and draw up an action plan.

→ Think positively. Pat yourself on the back when you overcome the urge to misuse food. If you have a minor slip, replay the scene in your mind and mentally rehearse a better resolution or outcome.

→ Remember that the only problem food solves is hunger.

How are you going to feel about losing weight three hours from now?

Proud of myself for making a good effort and getting closer to my goal!

If you listened to the second, more positive voice, give yourself a round of applause: You chose empowerment over giving in to a moment of weakness. It's only going to get better from here.

Just think how much more in control you'll be the next time you are reaching for an indulgent quick fix. By understanding the reasons behind your cravings, your pragmatic self will prevail.

WHAT'S YOUR CRAVING?

Cravings seduce us into misusing the worst types of food. None of my clients come in because they are addicted to crudités and fresh fruit. Their vices may seem trite: macaroni and cheese, tortilla chips, doughnuts, chocolate pudding. Yet their overreliance on foods loaded with fat and sugar can have devastating consequences.

Science is helping us better understand food cravings, those "gotta have it" urges set off by hunger, stress, particular places, or simply the sight and smell of something we find pleasurable. Research suggests the neuronal connections between food and behavior are made through life experiences. Our cravings may follow familiar, predictable, recurring patterns. I might crave my grandmother's chicken soup when I'm sad, always celebrate with cake, or grab salty snacks when I watch a movie because that's the pattern I have instilled in myself.

At Tufts University, researchers found that the most commonly craved foods among people on a calorie-restricted diet were foods high in both sugar and fat, such as chocolate, and foods high in salt, like chips and French fries. "What is commonly called carbohydrate addiction should probably be relabeled as calorie addiction," concluded Dr. Susan Roberts, the study's corresponding author.

Cravings don't necessarily go away during dieting, but on the Miracle Carb Diet, you have plenty of healthy alternatives to quell them without sacrificing flavor or the satisfaction of feeling full.

Fatty Foods and Carbs

Many people crave fatty foods because they taste good and have a pleasing texture and aroma. Butter, oil, lard, and margarine all are used frequently to add flavor to a wide variety of foods. That inclination goes way back. Evolution has hardwired your body to prefer fatty, high-calorie foods because they'll give you more energy for a longer period of time, which was a matter of survival back when we were cavemen living off of whatever we could hunt or gather while trying to survive in a dangerous world.

Many people find fatty foods comforting when they're bored, stressed, or upset. Sometimes it's because they're like familiar old friends who remind us of better times—it's not just the chocolate chip cookie you want, it's the coziness of your mom making them for you after school and the happiness you felt when you walked through the door and smelled them baking.

Fatty foods can be a pleasant distraction from your problems. Your body takes longer to burn the calories found in fatty foods, which can stabilize blood sugar levels to soothe feelings of anxiety and moodiness. Many fatty foods also contain tryptophan, an essential amino acid. Your brain uses tryptophan to produce serotonin, the neurotransmitter responsible for feelings of happiness and well-being. Serotonin also helps ease feelings of anxiety. Tryptophan overload at the Thanksgiving table is what makes us bliss-out in a turkey coma after the feast.

Cravings for fatty foods may also largely be a matter of habit. People often experience food cravings because they're accustomed to eating certain things in certain situations or in response to certain emotional cues (think pints of ice cream eaten straight from the carton and bad breakups, and you'll get the picture).

Sugar Cravings

Sugary foods can also provide sweet relief from negative feelings, because sugar raises your serotonin levels, which in turn induces brief feelings of happiness. You experience a sugar rush, and that brief release may be what you're yearning for if you find yourself craving sugar when you're unhappy or even bored. Like fatty foods, sugar cravings can occur by sheer force of habit. If you're used to having dessert after dinner, and you cut that out of your routine, you may go through a transition period of not merely missing your sugar hit but actually craving it. Your body will soon readjust, though, and definitely thank you for it later!

Salty Cravings

Some studies have traced salt cravings in women to a deficiency in calcium, potassium, or iron in low-calcium diets. One theory is that sodium temporarily increases calcium levels in the blood, tricking the body into thinking that there is no deficiency.

Chocoholics

You may reach for that chocolate bar because the flavor makes you swoon, but if you can't resist it, that may be the serotonin talking again. Chocolate is basically an antidepressant in dessert form that your body instinctively seeks out when your happy chemicals are bottoming out and you need a quick lift.

Crunchy, Crispy, Cold, and Creamy

If the sound of a potato chip bag opening makes you giddy, you probably fall into the category of cravers who are seeking out certain foods not just for their taste but for their texture. A bag of baby carrots can do the job if you need some serious crunching to decompress after a stressful day. Does the cold creaminess of ice cream comfort you post-breakup? Curl up on the sofa with a chilled cup of sugar-free pudding instead.

Now that you understand why and when you're most likely to overeat, you also see why excuses, not emotions, are to blame for keeping you in that vulnerable place for so long. Emotions are a vital part of our existence. We're entitled to feel whatever we feel, for whatever reason. But excuses aren't vital to our existence. They don't make us wiser, stronger, or more lovable. Or thinner. All they do is make us feel guilty.

From now on, food doesn't get to have control over your life. You do. *When the fork is in your hand, you are the one in control.* You decide when the benefits outweigh the sacrifices. You know already that you shouldn't be eating little pigs in a blanket. But guess what you're about to find out?

You'll never regret *not* eating them.

5

TRIGGERS AND TEMPTATIONS

O h, c'mon, just a little won't hurt! You've been so good, and you're looking great! What are you afraid of? You can afford to treat yourself; you can just make up for it tomorrow.

Anyone who has ever tried to lose weight is all too familiar with the voice of temptation. Sometimes the words come from the mouth of your insistent sister-in-law at the Christmas table or from a fun-loving non-dieter on a girls' night out. Or maybe you're just hearing that wheedling little voice inside your own head. Whatever the source may be, the voice of temptation is a force to be reckoned with. Face it, everyday life can seem like an obstacle course, especially when you're trying to lose weight and change your eating habits. Accept the fact that you can't handle each day and every situation perfectly—your best intentions and best-laid plans may not always be enough to keep you on track. That said, if you are serious about making this diet work its miracle, you have to aim high: Embrace your resolve to succeed and then live by it.

The principles behind the F-Factor plan are yours for a lifetime. And your commitment will pay off—I promise you that. Your job is to trust the knowledge and skills the F-Factor gives you to deal with hurdles both expected and unexpected. Remember, the changes you are making are not short term. It's time to break out of the old mind-set that dieting to lose weight is temporary, only in effect until you reach your goal.

At the end of the day, we all know we should be eating apples instead of French fries. Ignorance is no excuse when you make a bad choice about what you put in your mouth. Physiological hunger has little to do with it. A lot of the time we eat not to quell a hunger pang but because we're anxious, bored, or lonely. Or food just happens to be around within easy reach. From our well-stocked cabinets and well-meaning loved ones, to profit-driven food marketers, supermarkets, and restaurants, the field of enablers is wide and ever-present for overeaters. It's not always easy to tune them all out, but you can stay in control. Temptations aren't put in our path to defeat us; they are there to prove how strong and resourceful we are. You can train and strengthen your willpower much as you would your muscles. You can learn to resist temptation. But doing so requires meeting it head-on. In this chapter, I'll show you how.

Throughout my many years of practice, I continually come across the same diet hurdles. I'm here to tell you that you are hardly alone in your struggle with your weight. The solutions that have worked for so many others will help you kick your weight problem, too. Notice that I said *kick*, not *try to kick.* That's because the Miracle Carb Diet is your plan A for losing weight. There's no need for a backup plan because the F-Factor way is to make it part of your normal, everyday life—for the rest of your life.

GET UP AND GET OUT

Learn how to deal with your vices. If going out and gorging are synonymous to you, stop for a minute and really think this through: You are not being invited to parties or casual get-togethers because you're a good eater! Furthermore, if there is one indisputable truth you need to hold fast to about the F-Factor approach, it should be that dieting does not have to mean deprivation. I know I'd hate to be stuck at home alone eating some frozen diet dinner while my friends were out enjoying happy hour on a

Friday night, and I'm sure you would, too. I want to show you how to be healthy, not how to be a hermit. In fact, there is evidence that socializing can even make you skinnier. Research from Ohio State University Medical Center found that mice living in a socially stimulating environment—in this case, busy cages with lots of other rodent pals—were more likely to go for a spin on a wheel or a run through a maze, and when they were fed high-fat diets, they were less likely than their socially isolated counterparts to become obese. In other words: Having lots of social interaction seems to push you to lead a more active lifestyle and may even help keep you from gaining weight when your diet changes for the worse.

So from now on, you're not going to feel like the odd mouse out just because you are trying to take off some weight. There's no reason to stop going to the movies just because the theater's concession stand is a caloric minefield. Nor are you going to fake the flu to avoid your friend's New Year's Eve party or your nephew's confirmation. You are going to keep living your life—and live it well, if not even better—because you'll be socializing and enjoying what you eat and drink all along the way.

My client Richard is an inspiring example of this. When Richard first came in, he weighed 290 pounds and needed to shed 90 pounds of it. Everything about his lifestyle made continued weight gain a certainty. His successful career demanded that he entertain on a daily basis, so his schedule revolved around fine dining, cocktails, and fancy social events. "My whole life was spent going from meal to meal," he recalled. At home, Richard's partner was overweight as well, and for years they'd shared their passion for food, whether it was pizza and fried chicken around the kitchen table or discovering exotic cuisines on vacations all over the world. In one of our early sessions, Richard half joked of his addiction to cake. "Cake is my downfall," he confessed. Richard wasn't a food addict in the clinical sense, but the way he was misusing food had him careening down a precarious path.

Today, Richard is doing great; he's lost 60 pounds and is on target for reaching his goal weight very soon. He says he's never felt better—or more in control of the way he eats. That's because the Miracle Carb Diet has given Richard a sensible framework for healthy eating. Before, he basically followed his whims and cravings; his hefty physique, he reckoned, was proof that he was living the good life. When he started Stage One of the Miracle Carb Diet, Richard cut out processed foods and simple carbs, replacing them with great-tasting high-fiber foods that rid him of hunger and sugar cravings. He continued to dine out and drink without missing a beat. At home, Richard turned his love of food into a passion for cooking creatively. "I discovered all these herbs and spices at the store that add terrific flavor to vegetables," he reported. Richard also has learned how to peruse a restaurant menu for healthy fare and how to eat socially without filling up on empty calories and fat. And he still enjoys a slice of cake now and then—as a treat. Becoming aware of your weaknesses is a big step toward getting control of your weight, but weaknesses are not limited to food. Situations may set you up to overeat without you even realizing what's happening.

PORTION DISTORTION

Researchers have found that many people eat more because their meals are served on a large plate. It's a fact that in the past thirty years, the standard plate size has grown 25 percent, to 12 inches. Eat off a plate about 2 inches smaller and you'll serve yourself 22 percent fewer calories per meal, which can mean a 2-pound weight loss in one month, according to Dr. Brian Wansink, director of Cornell University's Food and Brand Lab and the author of *Mindless Eating: Why We Eat More than We Think.*

Proper portions can look skimpy served on a 12-inch plate, but put it on a 10-inch salad plate, and the same serving will look generous. Noshing snacks directly from the package can also distort our perception of serving size: One serving of potato chips is about ten chips, but it's hard to stop there if the bag is in your lap and an engrossing show is on TV.

Family-style dining can wreak havoc on your diet no matter what size plate you're using. It's easy to eat considerably more when food is served on platters and in bowls, which invite second and third helpings. Think about it: You'll be eating like it's a holiday every day if your dinners are served family style. Avoid this trap by preportioning your meals before you sit down at the table.

There's a knack to ordering well at a restaurant. First rule of thumb: Be yourself. Your personality, your great sense of humor, your wit and warmth—these qualities are what your tablemates want from you. Second rule: Don't feel compelled to explain yourself or apologize for not diving into that antipasto platter someone ordered for the table. Third: Ignore the group psychology at the table. Behavioral psychologists have found that if the first person to order is a big eater and drinker, the rest will follow suit. You don't have to. Instead, dig into the fun of catching up with your friends. Isn't that why all of you got together anyway?

Fill your heart, not your plate!

ATTITUDE ADJUSTMENT

I've counseled thousands of people over the years who truly struggle with their weight. It's heartbreaking when we make great strides in changing food choices and eating habits, only to see our efforts dashed by a lack of sustained commitment. I've never had a client gain back weight because of laziness. More often, after fighting the good fight, they throw in the towel and accept a lower standard for themselves. Why?

The internal argument goes something like this: *I have a beautiful family, everyone's healthy. I have a job I like and plenty of friends and a nice home. If I want to have more, won't God just think I'm greedy and ungrateful? I'm vain for wanting to be thin, right? Life is never perfect, so why am I striving for perfection?*

If I could only hit a delete button and erase that kind of thought process for you! Anything worth having in this life is worth working for, and that includes some of the most precious things we can have, like good health, high self-esteem, and great quality of life. We do ourselves a terrible disservice if we accept being overweight as our fate. I don't believe that the temptations are put in our paths to take us down; I think they are there to prove how strong and resourceful we really are. Losing weight is like holding down a job. It requires the same commitment to excellence day in and day out. And it takes the same level of nurturing one puts into raising families, advancing careers, and maintaining friendships. Succeeding at weight control is partly physiological and partly psychological. That's why the F-Factor way is as much about maintaining a positive outlook as it is about food choices.

Weight loss is serious, of course, but we need to keep a sense of humor in the face of challenges that we're bound to meet just going about our daily lives. I love the story my client Miriam told me. Miriam felt triumphant after a dinner party where the hostess pressured her to devour the mound of mushroom risotto heaped on her plate. "I spent half the afternoon making it from scratch. You won't taste a better risotto outside of Florence. I know you'll agree," the hostess boasted, glaring pointedly at Miriam's full plate. Not wanting to appear rude or indifferent, Miriam managed a few bites before artfully moving the rest to the edges, oohing and aahing on cue. "It made me feel like a naughty child," she admitted, but she gave herself well-deserved praise for handling such a tricky situation.

Miriam had in fact achieved an important milestone on her journey to lasting slimness: She had not allowed fear or embarrassment or ridicule to weaken her resolve. Often a person who is struggling with his or her weight also struggles with shame and self-doubt. When we feel bad about ourselves, the last thing we want to do is stand out, so we go along with the flow even though that tack usually proves self-defeating.

I know this from experience, having gained almost 25 pounds within six months of moving in with my husband. Glenn ate whatever he wanted and had no problem maintaining his lean, athletic build. For me, an extra slice of pizza or a beer on Saturday night eventually showed up somewhere on my slight five-foot-five frame. Instead of slipping into pretty lingerie at night, soon I was retiring in pajama bottoms and an oversize T-shirt. My friends wondered why I rarely went out. Little did they know that I'd outgrown most of my wardrobe; for me the idea of going out on the town was mortifying.

What advice would I have given myself back then? "Get off your butt and go out!" That's right. I firmly believe the best thing an unhappily overweight person can do is learn to get things right out in the real world. Learning how to dine fearlessly and deliciously can be incredibly empowering, because it puts you squarely in the driver's seat where you belong.

THINK THIN

Slim people go to parties, eat out, and handle stress without packing on the pounds. It's not because they are genetically blessed; it's because they've trained themselves on how to handle these situations.

Why not imagine yourself as a slender person going out for a wonderful meal? Be aware of what you put in your mouth from the moment you sit down. Order a drink or a glass of water, and wave away the bread basket. Choose a broth-based soup or leafy salad with dressing on the side and no croutons for an appetizer, and don't rush. Know before the entrée comes that you'll be eating only half; savor each bite slowly and consciously. Dessert, if ordered at all, is shared or just sampled. When this slender person—you—gets up from the table, you'll feel happy and satisfied. Not stuffed or tired or racked by guilt.

Adopting the mind-set of a thin person may also require you to change negative thought patterns. Your thoughts affect your emotions and your emotions can dictate behaviors. Thinking like a pessimist or defeatist is bound to create a self-fulfilling prophecy. So your first task is to stop thinking of your weight in black-and-white extremes. Stop baiting yourself with emphatic phrases that begin with *I should*, as in "*I should* be a size 4." If you have a fair amount of weight to lose, wouldn't it be more motivating to set interim goals and celebrate when you achieve them? And don't let past disappointments keep you from moving forward. You can't change history, but you can make positive choices that shape who you are today and tomorrow. Are your choices about eating and exercise different from those of someone who's trim and fit? How might they be the same? This is where journaling comes in. It helps you devise your personal game book for slimming success.

Remember, the reason we journal is that it reveals the details and patterns about how we eat. The Miracle Carb meal plans presented in Stages One through Three provide a proven framework for eating foods that are nourishing, satisfying, and conducive to weight loss. Fitting the F-Factor approach to your tastes and lifestyle is up to you. As you come to appreciate how much you are getting from that bowl of high-fiber cereal and berries, chances are you won't miss your old doughnut and double latte routine very much. Nor will you see the logic you once did in skipping lunch to leave more room for a great big dinner.

Journaling is much more than an accounting of food. It's where you'll see how your habits and emotions influence your food choices—and affect your weight. Through journaling, you will learn to take the reins of your diet and confidently stay the course.

FOILED AGAIN: HOW TO OUTSMART SABOTEURS

Never forget the power of two simple words: *No thanks*. You are not obligated to tack on any excuses, apologies, or elaborate explanations. But for more complicated situations, here are some troubleshooting tips.

Food Pushers

Some, like your Italian grandmother, may be doing it to show their love. If that's the case, let them be enablers, but enlist them in a better cause—keeping you healthy. Ask Grandma if she has a great veggie soup recipe, or better yet, offer to teach her one of your new F-Factor recipes! If someone is just proud of their culinary creation and eager for you to enjoy it, feed their ego instead of your belly by gushing over how beautiful the dish is or how wonderful it smells. Say you have no room for it now but would love to take a piece home for later—then you're in control of making sure later never happens.

But food pushers aren't always acting out of love. If you're getting negative remarks or pressure from a friend who is also overweight, he or she may be feeling anxious or threatened by your commitment to change. Undermining you and keeping you within the ranks of the overweight status quo is a way to avoid dealing with their own weight issues. You're not responsible for their feelings, but you are responsible for your reaction to this kind of pressure or negativity. If you don't feel like you can stand your ground, or discuss this openly with your friend, then step away.

Healthy Halo

Clever marketing can lull us into thinking we are eating more healthfully than we really are. The USDA found that diners ordering the "health-conscious" choices on restaurant menus usually failed to consider the average 443 calories added on with each side dish (and some popular chains include two free sides with each meal!). There's a similar halo effect in the grocery aisles with foods billed as natural, low fat, and organic. Many of these still contain a lot of calories, so the only way to know what you are eating is to read nutrition labels. You'll be surprised when you check out the labels of many fat-free foods and discover they actually have more calories than their full-fat versions. That's because sugar and other quick-digesting simple carbs are being used to make up for fatty ingredients. These foods can throw your blood sugar level out of whack and cause you to feel even hungrier soon after you finish eating them.

Drinking Calories

It's no secret that soft drinks and fruit drinks can pack a lot of calories. What you may not realize is that many of the beverages now being marketed as "healthy alternatives" aren't a whole lot better. To prove it, look no further than the nutrition label on a carton of fruit juice or a bottle of flavored iced tea or smoothie. The ingredients that make them tasty can also make them fattening. And you might assume that a carton or bottle is a single serving when it's probably two or even more. Think before you drink and check the nutrition label to avoid products high in calories and scant in nutrition. For quenching thirst you won't do any better than pure water. If you are choosing a fruit or vegetable drink because it promises a vitamin boost, you'll get far more nutrition by going directly to the source and eating the whole fruit or vegetable.

Big Eaters

Go out to dinner with big eaters and it's easy to become part of the pack. This is where knowledge gives you power. Ordering strategically from the moment you sit down lets you enjoy yourself while sticking to your eating plan. In fact, unless you tell your fellow diners that you are watching your weight, no one will know judging by what you drink and eat. On the Miracle Carb Diet, you'll be hard-pressed to find a restaurant that lacks in suitable choices.

Danger Zones

At work, if you know that the leftover pastries from the ten A.M. meeting are always in the conference room, stay away from that room. Take a different route to the elevator. If the sight of pizza being made in the window of the corner pizzeria makes you salivate, walk on the opposite side of the street. Pack your own snacks for your son's football game so you're not tempted by the concession stand.

THE SOCIAL SCENE

Making the most out of parties and staying on track when you're trying to lose weight takes a bit of premeditation. You can set yourself up for success with a few of my favorite little tricks.

- When scouring your closet for the perfect dinner outfit, look for clothes that are tailored and even perhaps a bit snug. It's much easier to overeat when you're wearing loose-fitting clothing. So try sticking to fitted pants or a tight skirt to discourage yourself from eating too much.
- Never go to a party hungry! Filling up before going out to eat is one of the best ways to help you lose or maintain your weight and keep your energy levels up. Going out to dinner on a full belly will allow you to avoid the nachos, to make smart choices, and to eat much less throughout the night.
- Being a social butterfly can help you stay on track as well. Cocktail hour can be a nightmare—cheese plates, sliders, and those adorable little quiches just begging you to come back for seconds! My advice for your next event is easy: Keeping your hands full always works. So does navigating your way to the shrimp cocktail, tuna tartare, and crudités.

- Finally, never skip buffet reconnaissance. Scan the tables before you choose what you are going to have.

QUICK TIPS FOR STAYING ON TRACK

- Nip a sweet craving by eating something sour. Feel an ice cream binge coming on? Bite into a pickle or sip some lemony water or tea.
- At the salad bar, fill your plate with fiber first, and save the high-calorie indulgences for your last stop. Build your plate by piling on the leafy greens first, then vegetables, and finish with just a tasting portion or two of fatty meats or creamy salad dressing.
- Drink a tall glass of water before a meal, and if you're grabbing a snack at a gas station or convenience store, grab a bottle of water as well. Open it and start drinking before you even get back into your car. Why? Because the water will create the feeling of fullness.
- Savor every bite. Try to actually think about the food that's in your mouth and what you enjoy about it—the freshness, or the pleasing texture, or the interesting blend of spices and flavorings. Eat the way a toddler does (minus the lack of manners!). Be amazed by food. Dawdle over it. People who eat at a slower pace feel satisfied eating less. Those who eat quickly are more apt to overeat; they're more likely to not only clean their plate but also habitually take second helpings.
- Snack strategically before a meal. A healthy pairing of carbs and protein, like high-fiber crackers with a wedge of light snack cheese, will stabilize your blood sugar, which in turn diminishes cravings and ravenous hunger.

HEALTHY CHOICES ON THE GO

- **Beware of Hidden Ingredients:** A turkey sandwich on wheat may sound healthy, but not so much if it's slathered with mayonnaise and topped with bacon. Condiments and extras alone can add 700–800 calories and more than 20 grams of fat to your "healthy" sandwich! If your only choices are premade, packaged sandwiches where you don't have the option of asking them to hold the mayo and extras, then look for a veggie option, or a lean protein such as turkey or chicken, with little or no mayo.

- **Fruit Never Fails:** Fresh fruit or fruit salads sold at many food stands are always a good, low-fat bet. Coffee shops offer bananas, and cups of fresh fruit salad can usually be found in the cooler case.

- **Go Nuts!** You can find packets of nuts and nut mixes everywhere these days, and the varieties are endless. There are spicy combinations with fiery wasabi, sweet mixes with dried fruit, raw nuts, dry-roasted nuts, yogurt-covered nuts—you name it, and a nut probably has it. Just remember that moderation is key. A single serving of nuts is 1 ounce and how many you get depends on which type of nut you choose. There are forty-nine pistachio kernels to a single serving, or you can have thirty peanuts, or twenty-three almonds.

- **Coffee Break:** If healthy food is nowhere in sight and your stomach is growling, grab a tall skim latte. The milk has some protein and calcium, and it may be enough to fill you up or tide you over.

- **Personal Picnic:** If you tend to go overboard with portions or mindless noshing, you're probably better off carrying your own premeasured snacks in sandwich baggies. Raw nuts, high-fiber bars or crackers, soy nuts, chopped vegetables, and bottled water are all good choices. You can keep a single 15-gram serving of approved carbs in a baggie. Some of my clients find it helpful to divvy a box of crackers or a bag of air-popped popcorn into separate 15-gram serving baggies as soon as they open the container, so the correct portions are always available. You're not likely to sit down and eat five baggies full of your favorite snack in one sitting, but you could easily consume five servings if you eat straight from the box or bag.

TIPS FOR MAKING A SLIMMER SALAD

Make Your Own: You know what you love most in a salad, so do it yourself and toss in some really good stuff, like hearts of palm, roasted peppers, kidney beans, edamame, albacore tuna, beets, etc.

Not Chopped: It takes longer to eat a big leafy salad than one that is finely chopped. The extra time spent eating allows your brain to catch on that you are full.

Dress for Success: Vinaigrettes contain oil and therefore more calories. Balsamic vinegar, delicious and just 5 calories per tablespoon, is a much better bet.

Add Healthy Crunch: Instead of croutons, top your salad with a tablespoon of slivered almonds, which have only 52 calories and contain fiber, protein, and heart-healthy fat.

MOVIE THEATER TIPS

Nothing spells temptation like the aroma of hot popcorn when you walk into a movie theater! Those self-serve tanks of "buttery flavor" (i.e., oil) don't help, either. Since childhood, we're all conditioned to associate the experience of going to a movie with popcorn, soda, and candy. A triple calorie bomb.

On average, a large tub of popcorn holds 20 cups and contains approximately 100 grams of fat—the equivalent of more than six fast-food burgers! With about 1,300 calories, that snack equals almost a full day's supply of calories for the average dieter. If you're thinking nachos with cheese wouldn't hurt—hey, it's dinner!—you're in for a 1,101-calorie surprise, complete with 59 grams of fat and 23.6 grams of protein. A hot dog on a bun with ketchup has 315 calories with 18.5 grams of fat and 10 grams of protein.

Bring healthy, preportioned snacks to the cinema so that you won't have to worry about munching on empty calories.

Stage One

- ☞ Diet soda or Crystal Light
- ☞ F-Factor Chai Tea "Latte" (chai tea with steamed soy or skim milk and Splenda)
- ☞ 1 cup of F-Factor Trail Mix (high-fiber cereal mixed with slivered almonds and raisins)
- ☞ 1 ounce of almonds or pistachios
- ☞ Sugar-free hard candies (up to 5)
- ☞ 1 bag of Brothers-All-Natural Fruit Crisps

Stage Two

- ☞ 1 F-Factor Bar
- ☞ 1 bar of HealthSmart Chocolite (candy or protein)
- ☞ 1 bag of Popchips or Chip'ins
- ☞ 1 mini bag of Orville Redenbacher SmartPop! (100 calories)
- ☞ 1 bag of Fiber Gourmet Lite Nacho Snacks Crackers
- ☞ Dry-roasted edamame
- ☞ Fruit (grapes, blueberries, clementine)
- ☞ Banana (counts as 2 fruits)

AIRPORT SURVIVAL KIT

Whether you're headed home for the holidays, taking off on a long-planned vacation, or traveling for business, being on the road can undo your best-laid eating and exercise plans. Airports in particular can be a diet disaster—cinnamon buns, buttery pretzels, and king-size bags of chips and candy abound.

The key to staying on track with your diet is planning ahead and always keeping healthy snacks stashed in your carry-on bag. Forgetting to pack healthy snacks can make high-calorie foods sold in the terminal very tempting, especially if your flight is delayed. Start your trip off right, with these simple recommendations.

Tips for Purchasing Food at Airports:

☞ Stay away from any sandwiches laden with heavy mayonnaise or bacon. Tuna and egg salad sandwiches are often very high in fat from mayonnaise. If available, opt for sandwiches with veggies and lean protein, such as turkey or chicken, with little to no mayonnaise. And there's no law that says you can't get the sandwich and just eat the lean protein without the mayo-sodden bread or bacon.

☞ Many delis and restaurants offer grilled chicken or a garden salad with dressing on the side, which are generally good picks.

☞ Airport food stands often sell yogurt. Choose low-fat, reduced-sugar versions. To add some crunch and fiber, bring individual portions of high-fiber cereal (put ½ cup servings into baggies) to sprinkle on yogurt.

☞ Fresh fruit cups can often be found in cooler cases and are always a good, low-fat bet. If you're heading home from a trip, grab one of the complimentary fresh apples many hotels now keep at the reception desk or in the breakfast room when you check out, and tuck it into your carry-on for later.

☞ Many airport stores sell large bags of nuts mixed with dried fruit. While nuts in moderation are great sources of heart-healthy fat, one serving may range from 130–160 calories and contain 13 grams of fat, and many bags contain as many as ten servings! If you tend to go overboard with portions, you would probably be better off bringing your own nuts in premeasured amounts. Small bags of almonds can also sometimes be found at the register at Starbucks and other coffee stands.

Some Portable Snack Options:

☞ Raw nuts (but keep the portions to about ¼ cup) and soy nuts

☞ Fresh or dried fruit

☞ Pretzels

☞ Low-sugar granola bars

☞ Low-fat energy bars

☞ Mini carrots

☞ Bottled water

Foods to Pack

You may find yourself in a terminal where no healthy food is available. Always come equipped with snacks on hand. The table below will give you snack ideas that are both convenient and nutritious. They are designed to provide you with some protein and fiber to keep you feeling full longer.

	Calories	Fat (g)	Sat. Fat (g)	Carbs (g)	Fiber (g)
Thomas' Light Multi-Grain English Muffin with 1 tablespoon peanut butter and 1 tablespoon sugar-free jelly	200	8	1	32	9
Glenny's Soy Crisps, lightly salted (1 bag)	140	3	0	18	3
Fiber One Cereal (½ cup portions)	60	1	0	25	14
Fiber One Bar Oats and Chocolate	140	4	1.5	29	9
Kashi Chewy Granola Bar Honey Almond Flax	140	5	.5	19	4
Raw veggies (1 cup of carrots, cucumber slices, bell peppers)	50	0	0	11	3
Medium apple	80	0	0	15	4
Medium banana	105	0	0	30	2
High-fiber crackers (per cracker)	12	0	0	7	5
Laughing Cow Light cheese (1 wedge)*	35	2	1	1	0
Bumble Bee Sensations Seasoned Tuna Medley Bowl Sundried Tomato & Basil	130	5	1	2	0

(continued)

	Calories	Fat (g)	Sat. Fat (g)	Carbs (g)	Fiber (g)
Almonds (1 ounce)	160	14	1	6	3
Pistachios (1 ounce)	160	13	1.5	7	3

* *Does not need to be refrigerated*

There's no denying that food plays a starring role in our world, and unless you live in a sealed biosphere in some desert, you're going to be bombarded by triggers and temptations on your way to becoming the slim, healthy person you dream of being. Remember that every small victory—the dessert you decline, the fifteen minutes you spend lifting weights instead of noshing in front of the TV—gets you that much closer to your greater goal.

It's not supposed to be easy. Anything worth having is worth working for, and you don't get the ideal body by taking the easy road!

6

RAISE YOUR GLASS

As a dietitian—and as someone who enjoys socializing over cocktails—I believe you can and should be able to drink moderately even if you are trying to lose weight. Alcohol needn't sabotage your diet, and it certainly isn't the reason why so many Americans are overweight. In Europe, where people enjoy wine and spirits at lunch and dinner, they don't have the incidence of obesity that Americans do.

In fact, a study published in the *Archives of Internal Medicine* found that light to moderate drinkers actually gain less weight than teetotalers over time, and they have a lower chance of becoming overweight or obese. I know this from experience working with my clients who consistently lose weight without abstaining from alcohol. Instead of asking them to cut out alcohol, I help them learn to drink a bit smarter by avoiding unnecessary calories.

Social drinking may be part of your lifestyle, whether you like to go out to clubs and restaurants on weekends, or you conduct business meetings over dinner, or you enjoy cooking and entertaining at home. Abstaining from alcohol just because you are on a diet would take something away from you that you'd miss. I don't recommend it because, feeling deprived can set you back far more than a glass of wine ever could.

How many times have you gone out to dinner with someone who immediately announces, "I'm not drinking, I'm on a diet!" and then proceeds to sip water while sponging up olive oil with her bread and orders a Caprese salad? A glass of wine has only 90 calories—far less than the bread soaked in olive oil with a whopping 360 calories or more, or 3–4 slices of fresh whole-milk mozzarella that will set you back 400 calories or more! Do the math and you can see why drinking alcohol in moderation won't cause weight gain.

For me and for many people I know, having a glass of wine with dinner or meeting up for an after-work drink adds to our overall quality of life. Sitting down at my favorite restaurant is not the time for me to say no to having cocktails for fear that they will ruin my diet. Since we know drinking in moderation doesn't cause weight gain, why give it up? The key to drinking and dieting is to be sensible and stay in control without feeling deprived. Some questions to ponder: Which will you enjoy more—alcohol or food? Are you happier with an appetizer, entrée, and a glass of wine, or will you be more satisfied having an appetizer with a small green salad and two or three glasses of wine? It's your choice, but know that you cannot have it both ways.

Might drinking alcohol potentially put you in an "Oh, why not?" frame of mind and lead you to eat or drink too much? If having a few drinks at happy hour lowers your inhibitions to the extent that you wind up gorging on the bar snacks, then plan ahead and eat a filling high-fiber snack beforehand. Then order a crudités platter with your drink and skip the complimentary bowl of nuts. After all, raw veggies are healthy and virtually calorie-free, whereas a few handfuls of roasted nuts can pack more than 200 calories, the equivalent of one and one-half lemon drop martinis! Make sure you sip water in between cocktails to prevent dehydration, or stick to one drink before switching to water or diet soda.

Keep in mind why you enjoy happy hour in the first place: to spend quality time with your friends —not to drink and eat too much. There's no reason alcohol should ever interfere with your having a great time. You can make this work.

One way to go easy at the bar is to order a less-caloric version of your usual drink. For example, order vodka, tequila, or other spirits with zero-calorie club soda and a splash of your favorite juice instead of 90-calorie tonic, or take a cue from the Europeans and have a wine spritzer (half wine, half club soda). And beware of mixed drinks. A margarita or any sugary cocktail can wind up being anywhere from 450–600 calories. Opt instead for tequila with a splash of juice and a wedge of lime, or ask for flavored vodka mixed with soda water.

Your best bet for low-cal drinking is wine and spirits, with each containing about 70 calories per drink. If mixed drinks are more your style, would you rather have two rum and Diet Cokes or one specialty cocktail, such as a cosmopolitan, for the same 140 calories? Again, the choice is yours.

For journaling, refer to the Miracle Carb Bible for carb and fiber content. All the current nutrition and health guidelines recommend a maximum of one drink a day for women and two for men. One drink equals 1.5 ounces (one shot) of 80-proof distilled spirits, 5 ounces (a little less than the size of a yogurt container) of wine, or 12 ounces of light beer. One slice of white bread has 15 grams of carbs—equal to one serving of carbohydrate. On the Miracle Carb Diet, we use a slice of white bread as a useful reference for comparing options (as you can see on page 146).

TIPS AND TRICKS FOR VACATIONS AND SOCIAL SITUATIONS

Vacation

Who doesn't love a refreshing drink while relaxing on a sunny beach? Vacation makes it easy to consume a lot of high calorie drinks, though, so pace yourself and choose wisely. Instead of tossing back a frosty margarita, mojito, daiquiri, or other sugary concoction, why not go instead for something lighter and equally potent, such as tequila with a splash of pineapple or grapefruit juice, or coconut rum with coconut water on the rocks. For

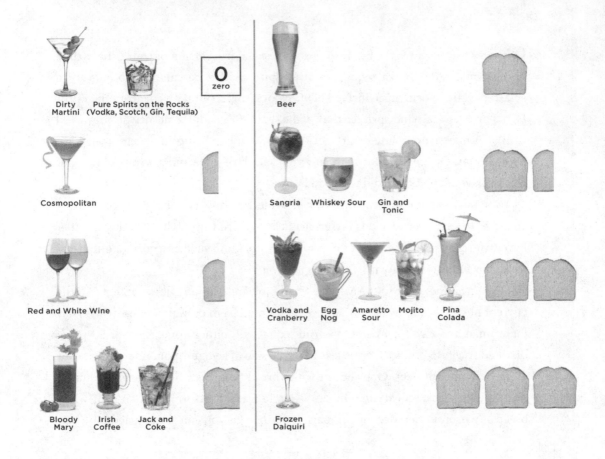

Dirty Martini • Pure Spirits on the Rocks (Vodka, Scotch, Gin, Tequila) • **O** zero • Beer

Cosmopolitan • Sangria • Whiskey Sour • Gin and Tonic

Red and White Wine • Vodka and Cranberry • Egg Nog • Amaretto Sour • Mojito • Pina Colada

Bloody Mary • Irish Coffee • Jack and Coke • Frozen Daiquiri

variety, you just can't beat drinks made with flavored vodkas, such as strawberry, mango, ruby red, blueberry, watermelon, raspberry, black cherry, green apple, or vanilla. My poolside favorites are passion fruit vodka with a splash of pineapple juice and green apple vodka with a splash of cranberry.

Events and Social Situations

Those drinks at the open bar may be free, but they aren't calorie-free. You can still live it up without drinking away a half-day's calories. Just beware those designer cocktails, because the mixes that make them sweet and colorful are probably laden with sugar. One green apple martini has about the same calories as two or three scotch and sodas. If you are satisfied having just one cocktail but don't want to seem like a party pooper, just switch to a glass of water or seltzer garnished with lemon or lime, and no one will be any the wiser.

Entertaining at Home

In your own home, you decide what drinks to serve your guests. Instead of tending bar, spend more time socializing by serving one cocktail for all from a pitcher, like sangria. True, a serving of traditional sangria weighs in at 130 calories and about 13 g of carbohydrates—equivalent to one slice of white bread! But you can cut this in half by making your sangria with diet ginger ale, wine, and club soda, garnished with fresh lemons and limes. Cut calories without sacrificing appearance or taste by using low-cal mixers such as diet soda and low-sugar juices, or try Crystal Light's sugar-free margarita, mojito, and appletini mixes. For more ideas, check out my F-Factor cocktail recipes at the end of Chapter 7.

HANGOVERS

Okay, so you partied a little too hearty last night and now you're feeling mighty queasy and your head is ready to explode. The reason you feel so terrible is that drinking too much alcohol left you dehydrated and suffering from low blood sugar (reactive hypoglycemia). Your first inclination may

> → If you wake up feeling nauseated, drink ginger tea with honey and lemon, which will help ease the nausea and settle your stomach.
> → Stick to vegetables and fruits the day after; they are rich in antioxidants, vitamins, and minerals that will help the body get back to normal. Tomatoes are a good source of vitamins A and C, beta-carotene, and the antioxidant lycopene, while bananas are good for replenishing electrolyte potassium.

be to reach for the greasiest, fattiest foods (fried eggs, home fries, a side of bacon, a stack of buttered toast), but won't that put a dent in your diet? Infinitely better: Drink plenty of water and eat fruit. The water will help flush your system and the sugars in the fruit will help raise your blood sugar to normal levels again.

Next time, to prevent a hangover, try eating before and while you drink. Food binds with certain impurities in alcohol, called congeners, and keeps them from being absorbed by your body. Eating high-fiber carbohydrates are your best bet, because they slow the absorption of alcohol. Things that speed up absorption and can cause a nasty hangover: sweet carbonated mixers and warm drinks like Irish coffee. Now I can't promise that you'll never again suffer a hangover, but by learning how to drink smarter, you can avoid the worst kind of hangover. My best tip: Pace yourself by alternating every alcoholic drink with a glass of water, and drink a small bottle of water before going to sleep.

BEST AND WORST COCKTAILS FOR DIETERS

Best

Gin and Diet Tonic, Vodka and Club Soda, and Rum and Diet Coke: It's a three-way tie with only 65 calories per 8-ounce glass! This is because when you drink a 1-ounce pour of most liquors and top them off with a calorie-free mixer, you have a drink that's pretty low in calories, no matter what the combination. Be mindful that many establishments generously pour 1.5-ounce shots into their drinks, so ask for a 1-ounce pour or a skimpy pour. Whether you choose gin, vodka, whiskey, or rum, top it off with a mixer that adds nothing: club soda, Diet Coke, or diet tonic water. Make them more exotic with flavor-infused alcohol, splashes of juice, or sugar-free syrups (though the latter two will add a few calories).

White Wine Spritzer: Make your wine order a wine spritzer and you'll automatically cut the calories in half. The concept of the spritzer is simple: white wine mixed in equal proportions with club soda. Depending on the wine you use, it can be refreshingly sweet or dry and only 50 calories per 5-ounce glass. And while some might think it's an atrocity to mix a nice Pinot Grigio with *anything*, it's your body, and if you prefer a spritzer to a beer gut, it's your prerogative. Make a spritzer prettier with a blush wine, or add a squeeze of orange or lime juice for oomph. However many you have, it'll be half the calories of regular wine.

Martini: Martinis are practically straight liquor, but shaken with ice and an aromatic splash of vermouth, they have a cocktail sensibility of 160 calories per 2.5-ounce glass. The taste can be strong for a drinker who likes sweeter drinks, and if that's you, order your martini made with infused liquor that adds flavor without added calories. Vanilla-flavored vodka makes a wonderful martini, but for something more daring, try one of the many brands of spicy pepper-infused liquors.

Mimosa: Half Champagne and half orange juice, mimosas are best when made with the freshest-squeezed juice imaginable and are only 75 calories per 4-ounce Champagne glass. Don't even worry about which Champagne. In all honesty, it doesn't matter. If it makes you happy to buy the expensive stuff, by all means, knock yourself out.

Kahlua and Coffee: The Starbucks coffee craze has gotten people thinking up crazy calorie-filled concoctions, but luckily, one of the old standbys of classic cocktails can fulfill your alcohol *and* your caffeine needs with substantially less calories at 91 calories per 6 ounces. Kahlua is the most famous brand of coffee-flavored liqueur, but any type will do, and even the best-brewed coffee still has *0* calories. With such a light drink, you can afford to add a bit of skim milk to make it creamy. You can enjoy this mixture in a steaming mug on a cool night, or ask your bartender to serve it iced in a tall glass. Iced Kahlua and coffee makes a stimulating, slimming drink on a hot summer day, and you'll see the results on the scale.

Worst

Margarita: If you're planning on ordering that margarita, you may want to think again. This one drink has about 750 calories and 56 grams of carbs. Substitute it with tequila on the rocks with a splash of lime.

LEAST CALORIC DRINKS—AT A GLANCE

	Calories	Carbs	Fiber
Bloody Mary	120	5	1
Red or white wine, 3.5 ounces	100	2	0
Distilled liquors (whiskey, gin, rum, vodka), 90 proof, 1 ounce	100	0	0
Gin/vodka and diet tonic	100	0	0
Rum and Diet Coke	100	0	0
Champagne	100	0	0
Low-carb beer	99	3	0
White wine spritzer	50	1	0

Long Island Iced Tea: This powerful cocktail has about 750 calories with 44 grams of carbs. Instead, try rum mixed with Diet Coke and topped with a slice of lime; it will save you more than 600 calories.

Piña Colada: Your piña colada will set you back about 650 calories and 90 grams of carbs. Opt for vanilla-flavored vodka and Diet Coke/Sprite and you'll save yourself about 500 calories.

Cosmopolitan: Although cosmos only have 150 calories and 10 grams of carbs, we all know how hard it is to stop at one. It may not have as many calories as the other drinks on our list, but you'll drink this one quicker and find yourself ordering it again. A great alternative is vodka with diet cranberry juice.

7

RECIPES

STAGE ONE

STAGE TWO

STAGE THREE

High-Fiber Cracker Crumb Conversions

1 tablespoon	$1/3$ cracker
$1/4$ cup crumbs	$1^1/2$ crackers
$1/3$ cup crumbs	2 crackers
$1/2$ cup crumbs	3 crackers
$2/3$ cup crumbs	4 crackers
1 cup crumbs	6 crackers

SAUCES

Many people equate healthy food with bland food. I'd have to agree that a plain piece of broiled fish just doesn't sound that appetizing. What's the remedy for the healthy-but-boring dilemma? Add delicious sauces that pack in flavor—not calories. It's important to choose your tomato sauce wisely, as many are loaded with added sugar and extra calories. Keep these go-to sauces in your arsenal to dress up any dish, no matter which stage of the Miracle Carb Diet you're in.

QUICK AND EASY TOMATO SAUCE

I have to admit, I have a thing for tomato sauce, so much so that I needed a recipe for a quick sauce that I can throw together in a pinch. From pasta to grilled chicken, I'll slather just about anything with the stuff. My recipe is low in calories and rich in antioxidants, so go ahead—sauce it up!

1 tablespoon olive oil

1 small onion, diced

2 cloves garlic, chopped

12 plum tomatoes, chopped

8 basil leaves, sliced

2 teaspoons salt

1 teaspoon pepper

- Heat the olive oil in a large skillet over medium-high heat. Add the onion and garlic.
- Sauté the onion and garlic, stirring until onions are soft and translucent, about 2 minutes.
- Add the chopped tomatoes, basil, salt, and pepper to the skillet, and continue to cook for about 3–5 minutes.

SERVES 4

The Miracle Carb Diet Nutritional Content for Journaling
Per serving: 0 g carbohydrate, 4 g fiber

Actual Nutritional Content

Per serving: 74 calories, 11 g carbohydrate, 4 g fiber, 2 g protein, 3 g total fat, .3 g sat. fat, 321 mg sodium

SLOW-SIMMERED MARINARA

Tomato sauce takes on a deliciously robust flavor when slowly simmered over a stove. Whenever I can find the time, I'm in my kitchen stirring up a big batch of this Italian standard. The aroma of vegetables and seasonings fills my kitchen with a fragrant smell right out of an Italian trattoria.

1 tablespoon olive oil

2 small onions, finely chopped

2 cloves garlic, minced

1 teaspoon dried oregano

2 stalks celery, finely chopped

2 carrots, peeled and finely chopped

½ teaspoon salt

½ teaspoon pepper

2 (32-ounce) cans crushed tomatoes

1 dried bay leaf

2 teaspoons dried basil

2 tablespoons fresh flat-leaf parsley, roughly chopped

- In a large pot, heat the oil over medium-high heat. Add the onions, garlic, and dried oregano, and sauté until the onions are translucent, about 5 minutes.
- Next, add the celery, carrots, salt, and pepper. Continue to sauté until the vegetables are soft, about 5 minutes.
- Add the crushed tomatoes, bay leaf, and basil. Reduce heat and simmer uncovered for 1 hour.
- Remove the bay leaf from the sauce, add the fresh flat-leaf parsley, and stir gently.
- You can either serve the sauce right away or it can be kept refrigerated for up to 1 week or frozen for 1 month.

SERVES 8

The Miracle Carb Diet Nutritional Content for Journaling
Per serving: 0 g carbohydrate, 3 g fiber

Actual Nutritional Content
Per serving: 64 calories, 12 g carbohydrate, 3 g fiber, 2 g protein, 2 g total
    fat, 0 g sat. fat, 375 mg sodium

HEARTY BOLOGNESE

*This hearty sauce is one of my absolute favorites. So much so that if you
walked into my kitchen, you just might find me having a spoonful of it on its
own! This sauce combines tomatoes, beef, and veggies and adds tons of flavor to any dish.*

1 teaspoon olive oil

1 medium onion, finely chopped

2 cloves garlic, minced

1 carrot, finely chopped

2 stalks celery, diced

1 pound extra-lean (90 percent)
    ground beef

1 cup cremini mushrooms,
    sliced

1¼ teaspoons dried oregano

1 (14-ounce) can crushed
    tomatoes

2 teaspoons Worcestershire
    sauce

½ cup beef stock or broth (or
    water)

2 teaspoons salt

½ tablespoon pepper

- Heat the olive oil in a large pot over medium-high heat.
- Sauté the onion, garlic, carrot, and celery until soft, about 5 minutes.
- Add the ground beef to the pot and cook, stirring continuously, for
  about 5–7 minutes, or until the ground beef has browned.
- Add the remaining ingredients. Reduce heat and simmer for about 30
  minutes, stirring occasionally.

SERVES 4

The Miracle Carb Diet Nutritional Content for Journaling
Per serving: 0 g carbohydrate, 18 g fiber

Actual Nutritional Content
Per serving: 245 calories, 13 g carbohydrate, 3 g fiber, 24 g protein, 10 g total
fat, 3 g sat. fat, 148 mg sodium

FRESH BASIL PESTO

This quick and easy pesto is a great change from red sauce. While tradi-
tional pesto recipes call for tons of calorie-laden oil, I've managed to reduce
the oil while maintaining the flavor. Keep in mind that the fresher the basil
you use, the better this sauce will be.

1½ cups basil leaves

2 tablespoons pine nuts, toasted

½ cup grated Parmesan cheese

2 cloves garlic, peeled and
   quartered

¾ teaspoon salt

½ teaspoon pepper

2 tablespoons fresh lemon juice

2 teaspoons olive oil

¼ cup low-sodium chicken
   broth

In a food processor or blender, puree the basil, pine nuts, Parmesan
cheese, garlic, salt, pepper, and lemon juice. Scrape the sides of the bowl
with a spatula, and then add the olive oil and chicken broth. Continue to
puree until smooth.

SERVES 8

The Miracle Carb Diet Nutritional Content for Journaling
Per serving: 0 g carbohydrate, 1.5 g fiber

Actual Nutritional Content
Per serving: 75 calories, 3 g carbohydrate, 2 g fiber, 4 g protein, 5 g total fat,
2 g sat. fat, 316 mg sodium

THAI PEANUT SAUCE

This spicy peanut sauce is absolutely addictive, and the good news is that you can have it from day one on the Miracle Carb Diet. It's perfect drizzled over noodles and vegetables, and it can also serve as a seemingly decadent dip.

3 tablespoons soy sauce

2 tablespoons rice or white wine vinegar

2 tablespoons nonnutritive sweetener

½ cup PB2, unprepared

½ cup water

1 teaspoon toasted sesame oil

1 teaspoon ginger, freshly peeled and grated

2 scallions, chopped

- In a saucepan, whisk together the soy sauce, vinegar, nonnutritive sweetener, PB2, water, toasted sesame oil, and ginger.
- Place on medium-high heat and bring to a simmer. Turn heat to low and continue to simmer for about 5 minutes, until the sauce has thickened. Turn off heat and allow to cool.
- Once the sauce has cooled to room temperature, add the scallions.

SERVES 4

The Miracle Carb Diet Nutritional Content for Journaling
Per serving: 0 g carbohydrate, 1 g fiber

Actual Nutritional Content
Per serving: 57 calories, 4 g carbohydrate, 1 g fiber, 2 g protein, 4 g total fat, .5 g sat. fat, 677 mg sodium

SOUPS

There is no food I love more than soup. Perhaps it's because I am half Colombian, and it's common in Latin America to have soup as a first course at lunch and dinner. Or perhaps it's because I am half Jewish, and my grandma's chicken soup makes me recall happy family holiday dinners. But most likely, it's because, as a registered dietitian, I know that soup is the secret to a trim waistline. Soups fill you up, leaving less room in your belly for anything else. Your mind sees a big bowl of soup and psychologically you assume you'll be full. And soup does take up a lot of space in your tummy, so you tend to eat less of the course that follows. The trick is to eat broth-based soups filled with vegetables and lean proteins. These five soups are Miracle Carb staples. These delicious soups are all low in fat and most have less than 100 calories per cup, so seconds aren't just allowed but recommended.

GRANDMA CLAIRE'S CHICKEN SOUP

My grandma Claire makes the best chicken soup. It is a family tradition to serve it at every Jewish holiday. I also make it whenever my kids catch a cold. It works every time!

1 pound boneless, skinless chicken breast or 12 boneless, skinless chicken tenders, cut into bite-size pieces

1 quart water

1 (32-ounce) can fat-free chicken broth

Fresh parsley

8 whole peppercorns

3 sprigs fresh dill

2 bay leaves

4 carrots, peeled and cut into halves

2 turnips, peeled and cut into halves

1 onion, chopped

4 stalks celery, cut into large pieces

1 package whole wheat egg noodles (optional)

1 tablespoon salt

½ tablespoon pepper

SPECIAL EQUIPMENT:

Cheesecloth

- In a large pot over medium-high heat, place the chicken pieces and pour in the water and chicken broth.
- Cut the cheesecloth into a large enough piece to fit all the herbs and spices. Place the parsley, peppercorns, dill, and bay leaves into the cheesecloth, and tie up into a little bundle. Add the bundle and the vegetables to the pot. Add salt and pepper.
- Bring to a boil, then reduce heat to low and simmer for 1 hour, uncovered. (Optional: You can make chicken noodle soup by adding whole wheat egg noodles.)
- Use a ladle to skim any fat that rises to the top of the soup and discard. Remove and discard the cheesecloth.
- Turn off heat, and carefully remove the chicken and vegetables. Place on a cutting board or plate and let cool. Once cooled, shred the chicken and cut up the vegetables into small pieces.
- Add the chicken and vegetables back to the soup, and heat to serve immediately.

SERVES 8

The Miracle Carb Diet Nutritional Content for Journaling
Per serving: 0 g carbohydrate, 3 g fiber

Actual Nutritional Content
Per serving: 95 calories, 10 g carbohydrate, 3 g fiber, 5 g protein, 4 g total fat, 1 g sat. fat, 633 mg sodium

GARDEN VEGETABLE SOUP

A piping hot bowl of vegetable soup is a delicious way to get in your veggies. I stir up a pot of this soup at the beginning of every week so that I have a satisfying meal on hand whenever hunger strikes.

Nonstick cooking spray

1 cup onion, chopped

2 cloves garlic, minced

2 cups fresh spinach

2 cups broccoli florets

2 cups mushrooms, quartered

2 cups cauliflower, cut into bite-size pieces

2 cups fresh tomatoes, chopped, or 1 (15-ounce) can plum tomatoes

1 cup celery, chopped

6 cups chicken or vegetable broth

1 teaspoon dried oregano

1 teaspoon dried basil

½ tablespoon salt

1 tablespoon pepper

¼ cup grated Parmesan cheese (optional)

- Place a large pot over high heat. Spray with nonstick cooking spray. Add the onion and sauté for 2 minutes. Add the garlic and sauté for 2 minutes more.
- Add the spinach, broccoli florets, mushrooms, cauliflower, tomatoes, and celery to the pot. Stir, then add the broth, dried herbs, salt, and pepper.
- Bring the mixture to a boil, then simmer for 25 minutes, or until vegetables are tender. Before serving, stir in the Parmesan cheese, if desired, into the soup.

SERVES 8

The Miracle Carb Diet Nutritional Content for Journaling
Per serving: 0 g carbohydrate, 3 g fiber

Actual Nutritional Content

Per serving: 56 calories, 9 g carbohydrate, 3 g fiber, 4 g protein, .1 g total fat, 0 g sat. fat, 546 mg sodium

CREAMY TOMATO BASIL SOUP

Nothing says comfort like a big bowl of homemade tomato soup. I like to top this with low-fat shredded cheddar or Parmesan cheese and add crackers for a crouton-like crunch.

Nonstick cooking spray

1½ cups onion, chopped

4 cups (about 4 large) tomatoes, peeled, seeded, and chopped

⅓ cup fresh basil leaves, chopped, plus more for garnish

2 teaspoons salt

½ tablespoon pepper

2 quarts chicken broth

½ cup fat-free half-and-half

- Heat a large pot over medium heat. Spray nonstick cooking spray to coat the pot. Add the onion and cook until tender.
- Mix in the tomatoes and chopped basil. Add salt and pepper. Pour in the chicken broth, reduce heat to low, and continue cooking for 15 minutes.
- Transfer the soup to a blender (or use an immersion hand blender), and blend until smooth. Return to the pot and bring to a boil.
- Reduce heat to low, and gradually mix in the half-and-half. Pour the soup through a strainer before serving. Garnish each serving with a basil leaf, or top with shredded low-fat cheddar or Parmesan cheese.

SERVES 8

The Miracle Carb Diet Nutritional Content for Journaling

Per serving: 1 g carbohydrate, 2 g fiber

Actual Nutritional Content

Per serving: 66 calories, 10 g carbohydrate, 2 g fiber, 4 g protein, 1 g total fat, .5 g sat. fat, 158 mg sodium

CHUNKY GAZPACHO

Although traditional gazpacho is pureed, my favorite gazpacho is a chunky version from the Golden Pear Cafe in the Hamptons. The Hamptons are filled with farmer's markets stocked with local veggies. Here is my take on this refreshing chilled soup.

1 green bell pepper, seeded and chopped fine

1 red bell pepper, seeded and chopped fine

3–4 tomatoes, skinned, seeded, and chopped fine

2 large cucumbers, peeled, seeded, and chopped fine

1 large bunch cilantro, chopped fine, plus more for garnish

1 large red onion, chopped fine

3 large cloves garlic, minced

1 tablespoon Tabasco Sauce or 2 jalapeño peppers, finely chopped

1 (46-ounce) can tomato juice

¼ cup olive oil

Juice of 3 limes (optional)

1 packet Splenda

Salt, to taste

1 teaspoon pepper

Mix all the ingredients together. Add salt and pepper and mix. Let chill or cure in the refrigerator overnight. When ready to serve, ladle into bowls and top each one with a cilantro leaf.

SERVES 6

The Miracle Carb Diet Nutritional Content for Journaling

Per serving: 0 g carbohydrate, 4.5 g fiber

Actual Nutritional Content

Per serving: 183 calories, 24 g carbohydrate, 4.5 g fiber, 4 g protein, 10 g total fat, 1 g sat. fat, 136 mg sodium

CAULIFLOWER SOUP

Trick your taste buds with a silky soup so smooth you'd swear it included cream. While cauliflower might be white, it's certainly not pale in terms of nutritional content. Its nutrients help strengthen the immune system and fight against certain forms of cancer.

1 (12-ounce) microwavable steamer bag cauliflower

½ cup grated Parmesan cheese

1 (32-ounce) carton chicken or vegetable broth

1 teaspoon salt

2 teaspoons pepper

- Microwave the cauliflower for an extra 2 minutes of what the instructions on the bag say (to make the cauliflower extra tender).
- Add the steamed cauliflower, Parmesan cheese, salt, and pepper to a food processor, and pulse until coarse and thick.
- Add the chicken or vegetable broth to the processor slowly, a little at a time, until it is the consistency of soup (or, for a side dish, use less broth and make "mashed potatoes").

SERVES 6

The Miracle Diet Nutritional Content for Journaling

Per serving: 0 g carbohydrate, 1 g fiber

Actual Nutritional Content

Per serving: 71 calories, 3 g carbohydrate, 1 g fiber, 6 g protein, 4 g total fat, 2 g sat. fat, 740 mg sodium

DRESSINGS

What's the number one saboteur for many diets? It's salad dressing. Lettuce and vegetables contain less than 25 calories per cup. Two tablespoons of Caesar salad dressing has 200 calories! Even heart-healthy olive oil packs in 135 calories per tablespoon and 15 grams of fat. Plus, most restaurants use at least ¼ cup of dressing on your salad! Stick with our tried and true F-Factor salad dressings to keep your salads dressed just right!

BALSAMIC VINAIGRETTE

Many people think they are making the waistline-friendly decision by ordering balsamic vinaigrette on their salads. However, a standard vinaigrette dressing recipe calls for oil—and lots of it. My vinaigrette recipe, on the other hand, packs in a lot more flavor than plain old vinegar and a lot less calories than classic vinaigrette!

1 teaspoon olive oil

2 tablespoons lemon juice

3 tablespoons balsamic vinegar

1 teaspoon mustard (optional)

1 sprig fresh rosemary, chopped

⅛ teaspoon red pepper flakes

In a small bowl, whisk together all the ingredients until combined. Serve over any of your favorite salads or use as a marinade for fish or chicken.

SERVES 2 (2 TABLESPOONS PER SERVING)

The Miracle Carb Diet Nutritional Content for Journaling
Per serving: 0 g carbohydrate, 0 g fiber

Actual Nutritional Content
Per serving: 50 calories, 2 g carbohydrate, 0 g fiber, 0 g protein, 4 g fat, 50 mg sodium

GREEN GODDESS

Want to give your standard salad some flair? This creamy dressing is just the thing to make any dish a little more heavenly. Sure, it's great on lettuce, but it's also delicious on poached salmon or as a tasty dip for crudités.

½ cup low-fat mayonnaise

¼ cup green onion, chopped

1 clove garlic, minced

2 tablespoons fresh parsley, chopped

2 tablespoons fresh chives, chopped

1 teaspoon fresh tarragon, chopped

1 tablespoon tarragon vinegar

1 tablespoon lemon juice

1 teaspoon salt

2 teaspoons pepper

Puree all the ingredients in a food processor until creamy and smooth.

SERVES 8 (2 TABLESPOONS PER SERVING)

The Miracle Carb Diet Nutritional Content for Journaling
Per serving: 0 g carbohydrate, 0 g fiber

Actual Nutritional Content
Per serving: 44 calories, 3 g carbohydrate, 0 g fiber, .6 g protein, 3 g total fat, .6 g sat. fat, 220 mg sodium

TAHINI DRESSING

Tahini is a Middle Eastern sauce made out of sesame seeds. It is often an ingredient in the ever-popular hummus and oh-so-fun-to-pronounce baba ghanoush. However, the sauce is so delicious that I like to dip veggies in it, or have some smeared on crackers.

2 cups water

½ cup fresh lemon juice

1 teaspoon ground cumin

1 tablespoon garlic, minced

1 tablespoon fresh basil, chopped

1 cup tahini

In a blender, combine all the ingredients (except the tahini) until smooth. Add the tahini slowly until the dressing is the desired consistency.

SERVES 24 (2 TABLESPOONS PER SERVING)

The Miracle Carb Diet Nutritional Content for Journaling
Per serving: 0 g carbohydrate, 1 g fiber

Actual Nutritional Content
Per serving: 60 calories, 2 g carbohydrate, 1 g fiber, 2 g protein, 5 g total fat, 1 g sat. fat, 11 mg sodium

GINGER DRESSING

The ginger dressing served at Japanese restaurants is often the best part of the meal! It is so hard to find versions in the grocery store that are not high in calories and fat. Try this low-calorie flavorful version and add it to a salad at home!

½ pound carrots, peeled and chopped

¼ cup rice vinegar

¼ cup water

3 tablespoons fresh ginger, peeled and minced

1 tablespoon garlic, minced

2 tablespoons onion, chopped

2 tablespoons lemon juice

2 tablespoons low-sodium soy sauce

1 teaspoon toasted sesame oil

1 tablespoon olive oil

1 teaspoon salt

2 teaspoons pepper

Puree all the ingredients in a food processor until creamy and smooth.

SERVES 12 (¼ CUP PER SERVING)

The Miracle Carb Diet Nutritional Content for Journaling
Per serving: 0 g carbohydrate, 2 g fiber

Actual Nutritional Content
Per serving: 38 calories, 6 g carbohydrate, 2 g fiber, 1 g protein, 1.6 g total
   fat, 1 g sat. fat, 119 mg sodium

FRESH HERB RANCH DRESSING

Who doesn't love going for a dip in a deliciously creamy side of ranch dress-
ing? The only problem is that just 2 tablespoons of the stuff packs in 140
calories and 14 grams of fat! Instead, go skinny-dipping with my version:
Fresh Herb Ranch Dressing.

½ cup nonfat buttermilk

½ cup nonfat Greek yogurt

½ cup light mayonnaise

1 tablespoon fresh chives, finely
   chopped

1 tablespoon fresh flat-leaf
   parsley, finely chopped

1 teaspoon garlic powder

½ teaspoon onion powder

1 teaspoon salt

1 tablespoon pepper,
   to taste

Place all the ingredients into a bowl and stir well. Keep chilled until ready
to use.

SERVES 12 (2 TABLESPOONS PER SERVING)

The Miracle Carb Diet Nutritional Content for Journaling
Per serving: 0 g carbohydrate, 0 g fiber

Actual Nutritional Content
Per serving: 20 calories, 2 g carbohydrate, 0 g fiber, 1 g protein, 1 g total fat,
   0 g sat. fat, 35 mg sodium

SALADS/DIPS/SPREADS

High-fiber crackers or veggies with dip can be a great healthy snack option. It's an easy way to ensure that you're getting the winning combination of protein and fiber. It can also be an easy way to overload on calories really fast. Many classic dips have fattening bases such as full-fat cheese, sour cream, or mayonnaise, and we all know how hard it is to stop after the first dip! Instead, get dipping with my lightened-up favorites. These recipes are perfect to serve at your next party, to bring to a friend's get-together to ensure a healthy option is on hand, or to simply have come snack time.

F-FACTOR CHOPPED SALAD

This classic salad is a staple in my home. It's so simple—there basically isn't anything to do besides rinse and chop to have a healthy and delicious salad in no time. Make it a meal by topping it off with grilled chicken or shrimp.

4 plum tomatoes, seeded and cut into bite-size pieces

1 small red bell pepper, seeded and cut into bite-size pieces

1 small yellow bell pepper, seeded and cut into bite-size pieces

1 small red onion, cut into bite-size pieces

2 cucumbers, peeled, seeded, and cut into bite-size pieces

2 stalks celery, cut into in bite-size pieces

2 (14-ounce) cans hearts of palm, drained and chopped

2 (14-ounce) cans artichoke hearts, drained and chopped

In a large bowl, add all the vegetables and mix together. Chill in refrigerator until ready to serve.

SERVES 8

The Miracle Carb Diet Nutritional Content for Journaling

Per serving: 0 g carbohydrate, 2 g fiber

Actual Nutritional Content

Per serving: 100 calories, 18 g carbohydrate, 2 g fiber, 11 g protein, 2 g total fat, 1 g sat. fat, 490 mg sodium

TUNA SALAD

Tuna fish has just 35 calories per ounce and is full of omega-3s, but mayo has 100 calories per tablespoon and 10 grams of fat. Instead, make the simple switch to a low-fat or fat-free mayonnaise for your tuna salad, which averages about 15 calories and 1 gram of fat per tablespoon.

1 large carrot, chopped

2 stalks celery, chopped

1 (6-ounce) can of light albacore tuna, drained

1 teaspoon lemon juice

1½ tablespoons light mayonnaise

High-fiber crackers (optional)

- In a food processor, add the carrot and celery. Pulse until minced.
- Add the drained tuna, lemon juice, and light mayonnaise. Pulse until blended.
- Serve with high-fiber crackers.

SERVES 2

The Miracle Carb Diet Nutritional Content for Journaling

Per serving: 0 g carbohydrate, 2 g fiber

Actual Nutritional Content

Per serving: 100 calories, 7 g carbohydrate, 2 g fiber, 11 g protein, 3 g total fat, .5 g sat. fat, 133 mg sodium

EGG WHITE SALAD

Egg salad is a lunchtime staple, but not always the healthiest option, with most recipes calling for whole egg yolks and at least a ½ cup of mayonnaise. Kiss the yolk good-bye and swap the mayo for Greek yogurt to save big on calories and fat—without anyone knowing the difference!

Nonstick cooking spray

1 large onion, chopped

1 (1-pound) bag frozen chopped spinach, thawed and squeezed dry with a paper towel

2 teaspoons salt

1 teaspoon pepper

1 dozen boiled egg whites, chopped

6 tablespoons nonfat Greek yogurt

1 teaspoon mustard powder

¼ teaspoon garlic powder

¼ teaspoon fresh dill weed, minced

- In a saucepan sprayed with nonstick cooking spray, sauté the onion over medium heat for about 5 minutes, until translucent. Add the spinach, salt, and pepper, and cook until heated through. Let cool.
- In a medium-size bowl, combine the remaining ingredients with the sautéed spinach and onion mixture.
- Mix thoroughly and refrigerate for 1 hour before serving to bring out all the flavors.

SERVES 6

The Miracle Diet Nutritional Content for Journaling
Per serving: 0 g carbohydrate, 2 g fiber

Actual Nutritional Content
Per serving: 83 calories, 9 g carbohydrate, 2 g fiber, 12 g protein, 0 g total fat, 0 g sat. fat, 216 mg sodium

CHICKEN SALAD SPREAD

This chicken salad has the smooth consistency of tuna fish, and it is perfect for those of you who don't like the smell or taste of canned tuna! You need a food processor for this recipe. If you don't have one, you can hand chop everything—it just won't be as smooth.

4 cups water

2 teaspoons salt

1 teaspoon black peppercorns

1 carrot, diced

4 stalks celery, diced fine

$\frac{1}{4}$ cup onion, diced

1 pound boneless, skinless
    chicken breast

$\frac{1}{2}$ cup Hellmann's Light
    Mayonnaise

$1\frac{1}{2}$ teaspoons pepper

- In a large pot, add the water, 1 teaspoon salt, peppercorns, carrot, celery, and onion. Turn the stove to medium-high heat until boiling.
- Reduce to a simmer and add the chicken. Cook the chicken for 10–15 minutes (test a piece by cutting it in half to see if it is no longer pink).
- Remove the chicken and dry on a paper-lined plate. Allow to cool.
- Strain the soup mixture, and place the vegetables in a food processor. Pulse until just diced. Transfer vegetables to a large bowl. Add the chicken to the food processor and pulse until the chicken resembles flaked tuna fish.
- Transfer the chicken salad to a large bowl, add the light mayonnaise, remaining salt, and pepper, and stir well to incorporate all the ingredients.

SERVES 8

The Miracle Carb Diet Nutritional Content for Journaling
Per serving: 0 g carbohydrate, 1 g fiber

Actual Nutritional Content
Per serving: 145 calories, 5 g carbohydrate, 1 g fiber, 9 g protein, 5 g total fat,
    11 g sat. fat, 775 mg sodium

GREEK YOGURT DIPS:
FRENCH ONION AND VEGGIE

Greek yogurts like Fage, Chobani, and Oikos contain about half the calories and fat and three times the protein than fattening sour cream, making it a much healthier choice as a base for your dips.

FRENCH ONION DIP

2 (6-ounce) containers fat-free
    plain Greek yogurt
1 packet onion dip mix
1 tablespoon low-fat mayonnaise

1–2 tablespoons water
1 box frozen chopped spinach,
    thawed and squeezed dry
    with a paper towel

Mix the Greek yogurt with the onion dip mix, low-fat mayonnaise, and 1–2 tablespoons water. Add the spinach to the yogurt mixture and mix well.

    SERVES 6

The Miracle Carb Diet Nutritional Content for Journaling
Per serving: 3 g carbohydrate, 1 g fiber

Actual Nutritional Content
Per serving: 62 calories, 5 g carbohydrate, 1 g fiber, 8 g protein, 1 g total fat, 0 g sat. fat, 298 mg sodium

VEGGIE DIP

2 (6-ounce) containers fat-free
    plain Greek yogurt
1 packet vegetable soup
    mix
1 tablespoon low-fat mayonnaise

1–2 tablespoons water
1 box frozen chopped spinach,
    thawed and squeezed dry
    with a paper towel

Mix the Greek yogurt with the vegetable soup mix, low-fat mayonnaise, and 1–2 tablespoons water. Add the chopped spinach to the yogurt mixture and mix well.

SERVES 6

The Miracle Carb Diet Nutritional Content for Journaling
Per serving: 3 g carbohydrate, 1 g fiber

Actual Nutritional Content
Per serving: 62 calories, 5 g carbohydrate, 1 g fiber, 8 g protein, 1 g total fat, 0 g sat. fat, 248 mg sodium

STAGE ONE

BREAKFASTS

SPINACH AND FETA EGG WHITE OMELET

Spinach pie is one of my favorite foods, but at 600 calories per serving, it's a dish that I don't often indulge in. That's why I love this omelet recipe. It combines all of my favorite ingredients in spinach pie and is a perfect healthy breakfast to enjoy any day of the week.

Nonstick cooking spray

½ Vidalia onion or 1 large sweet onion, chopped

1 (10-ounce) package frozen chopped spinach, thawed and squeezed dry with a paper towel

1 dozen egg whites

1 teaspoon salt

2 teaspoons pepper

4 ounces low-fat feta cheese

2 high-fiber crackers (optional)

- Spray a skillet with nonstick cooking spray and heat over medium-low heat.
- Add the onion and sauté until translucent, about 3 minutes.
- Add the spinach and cook until spinach is warm. Transfer the spinach and onion mixture to a bowl and set aside.
- Season the egg whites with salt and pepper, and beat vigorously with a fork. Pour the egg whites into the skillet and gently stir until it begins to scramble.
- Sprinkle the feta cheese over the top, and then add the spinach and onions. Once the eggs are almost set, fold the omelet in half. Serve with high-fiber crackers, if desired.

SERVES 4

The Miracle Carb Diet Nutritional Content for Journaling
Per serving: 0 g carbohydrate, 2.5 g fiber

Nutritional Content

Per serving: 114 calories, 7 g carbohydrate, 3 g fiber, 14 g protein, 3 g total
fat, 1 g sat. fat, 368 mg sodium

MINI SPINACH AND HAM FRITTATAS

*If I'm hosting a brunch, you can bet I'll be serving these mini frittatas.
This mini egg dish makes it look like you slaved away in the kitchen
for hours, but it's actually oh-so-easy to whip up. Feel free to use any
of your favorite non-starchy vegetables in this recipe. These frittatas
are so delicious that you might just find yourself throwing a lot more
brunches!*

Nonstick cooking spray

2 (4-ounce) cartons frozen egg
  substitute, defrosted

½ cup reduced-fat milk

½ teaspoon pepper

⅛ teaspoon salt

4 ounces thinly sliced ham,
  Canadian bacon, or turkey,
  chopped

1 cup frozen chopped spinach or
  broccoli, thawed and
  squeezed dry with a paper
  towel

⅓ cup grated Parmesan or
  shredded mozzarella cheese

2 tablespoons fresh basil,
  chopped

SPECIAL EQUIPMENT:

12-cup muffin tin

- Preheat the oven to 375 °F. Spray the muffin tin with nonstick cooking
  spray and set aside.
- Whisk together the egg substitute, milk, pepper, and salt in a
  large bowl until thoroughly blended. Stir in the remaining ingredients.
- Fill the prepared muffin cups almost to the top with the egg mixture,

and bake until they puff up and just begin to set in the center, about 8–10 minutes.

- Using a rubber spatula, loosen the frittatas from the muffin cups and slide them onto a platter.
- Serve or wrap individually and keep in fridge. To reheat, microwave for 1 minute.

SERVES 12

The Miracle Carb Diet Nutritional Content for Journaling
Per serving: 1 g carbohydrate, .5 g fiber

Actual Nutritional Content
Per serving: 62 calories, 2 g carbohydrate, .5 g fiber, 6 g protein, 3 g total fat, 1 g sat. fat, 111 mg sodium

"BAGEL" AND LOX

As a New Yorker, I love my bagels, but did you know that just one bagel is the equivalent of seven slices of white bread? That's 560 calories (before the schmear) and 105 carbs! My take on a New York City bagel saves you 360 calories and 97 grams of carbs. Enjoy the better bagel.

4 ounces low-fat cream cheese	1 tablespoon fresh dill, minced
1 tablespoon Worcestershire sauce	¼ teaspoon salt
1 tablespoon green onion, chopped	¼ teaspoon pepper
1 tablespoon freshly squeezed lemon juice	3 ounces smoked salmon, minced
	2 high-fiber crackers (optional)

- Cream the cream cheese in an electric mixer fitted with a paddle attachment until just smooth.

- Add the Worcestershire sauce, green onion, lemon juice, dill, salt, and pepper, and mix.
- Add the smoked salmon, mix well, and chill.

SERVES 2

The Miracle Carb Diet Nutritional Content for Journaling
Per serving: 1 g carbohydrate, 0 g fiber

Actual Nutritional Content
Per serving: 200 calories, 8 g carbohydrate, 0 g fiber, 13 g protein, 11 g total fat, 5 g sat. fat, 660 mg sodium

TROPICAL FRUIT PARFAIT

Don't fall for the health halo; a restaurant fruit and yogurt parfait may not be as healthy as you think. Some have more sugar than two Krispy Kreme doughnuts! My recipe gives you the perfect light and sweet breakfast that won't weigh you down.

1 (6-ounce) container fat-free plain Greek yogurt
1 packet nonnutritive sweetener
¼ teaspoon almond extract
1 tablespoon slivered almonds
¼ cup (about ½) kiwi, chopped
¼ cup pineapple, chopped
¼ cup papaya, chopped
⅓ cup Kellogg's All-Bran Bran Buds

Mix the Greek yogurt with the nonnutritive sweetener and almond extract. Stir in the slivered almonds. Top with kiwi, pineapple, and papaya. Sprinkle with Kellogg's All-Bran Bran Buds.

SERVES 1

The Miracle Carb Diet Nutritional Content for Journaling
Per serving: 14 g carbohydrate, 17 g fiber

Actual Nutritional Content

Per serving: 200 calories, 20 g carbohydrate, 5 g fiber, 17 g protein, 6 g fat, 1 g sat. fat, 96 mg sodium

HOT CEREAL WITH VANILLA DRIZZLE

Start your morning off right by digging into a warm and filling bowl of hot cereal. This breakfast warms your tummy and keeps it full, too! The Vanilla Drizzle adds a delicious touch of sweetness. Talk about a good morning!

⅓ cup Kellogg's All-Bran Bran Buds

¼ cup Unsweetened Vanilla Almond Breeze

FOR THE VANILLA DRIZZLE:

½ cup fat-free Greek yogurt

½ teaspoon vanilla extract

¼ teaspoon cinnamon

1 packet nonnutritive sweetener

- Combine the cereal and almond milk in a microwavable bowl. Microwave on high to taste: 30 seconds for a *big* crunch; 60 seconds for a little crunch. If too thick, add a little extra almond milk to thin it out.
- In a small bowl, combine all the ingredients for the vanilla drizzle. Add a little water to thin it out. Stir until mixed well and drizzle over the hot cereal.

SERVES 1

The Miracle Carb Diet Nutritional Content for Journaling

Per serving: 39 g carbohydrate, 15 g fiber

Actual Nutritional Content

Per serving: 235 calories, 46 g carbohydrate, 15 g fiber, 21 g protein, 1 g total fat, 0 g sat. fat, 271 mg sodium

SALADS AND STARTERS

CALIFORNIA ROLL SALAD

Sushi is typically one of those foods best left to the experts to create. If you don't know what you're doing, those little rolls can quickly turn into one big raw-fish-and-rice mess. That's why I came up with this sushi salad—you get all the great taste elements of a California roll, no rolling required.

6 ounces imitation crabmeat

½ cucumber, diced

¼ avocado, diced

1 cup baby spinach

FOR THE DRESSING:

2 tablespoons fat-free
   Greek yogurt

1 tablespoon low-fat mayonnaise

½ teaspoon wasabi powder

1 tablespoon fresh lime juice

½ teaspoon salt

½ green onion, sliced, for
   garnish

- Mix the crabmeat, cucumber, and avocado together, and place on a bed of baby spinach leaves.
- Mix the dressing ingredients together until well combined. Spoon the dressing over the salad.
- Sprinkle the green onions on top of the salad, and serve.

   SERVES 2

The Miracle Carb Diet Nutritional Content for Journaling
Per serving: 0 g carbohydrate, 4 g fiber

Actual Nutritional Content
Per serving without dressing: 160 calories, 5 g carbohydrate, 4 g fiber, 19 g protein, 8 g fat, 1 g sat. fat, 495 mg sodium
Per serving with dressing: 195 calories, 7 g carbohydrate, 4 g fiber, 20 g protein, 9 g fat, 1.5 g sat. fat, 927 mg sodium

TUNA TARTARE OVER MIXED GREENS

Whenever I'm dining out and tuna tartare is on the menu, chances are I'll be ordering it. It's high in protein, low in calories, and big on flavor—what's not to love? My recipe takes this seemingly simple starter and turns it into an absolute standout.

1½ teaspoons wasabi powder

1 tablespoon water

3 tablespoons reduced-sodium (light) soy sauce

3 tablespoons seasoned rice wine vinegar

1 pound fresh tuna, trimmed and cut into ⅛-inch dice

1 ripe Hass avocado, peeled and diced

1 teaspoon salt

2 teaspoons pepper

3 cups mixed lettuce greens

- In a large bowl, add the wasabi powder and water. Use a whisk to make a smooth paste.
- Next, whisk in the soy sauce and seasoned rice wine vinegar.
- Gently fold the diced tuna, avocado, salt, and pepper into the wasabi mixture using a large spoon until all ingredients are well combined.
- To serve, place ½ cup of lettuce down on each plate, and top with ½ cup of tuna tartare.

SERVES 6

The Miracle Carb Diet Nutritional Content for Journaling
Per serving: 0 g carbohydrate, 2 g fiber

Actual Nutritional Content
Per serving: 225 calories, 5 g carbohydrate, 2 g fiber, 21 g protein, 4 g fat, 0 g sat. fat, 316 mg sodium

ASIAN COLESLAW WITH
SHREDDED CHICKEN

I'm not typically a coleslaw girl. Shredded lettuce with mayo? No thank you. Luckily, this is not your typical coleslaw. This Asian-inspired dish uses rice vinegar as a base and packs in a delicious crunch that creates an addicting twist on basic slaw. Just one bite is all you need to get hooked.

Nonstick cooking spray

1 pound chicken breast, thinly sliced

FOR THE DRESSING:

3 tablespoons rice vinegar

1 tablespoon vegetable oil

4 tablespoons PB2

2 tablespoons water

2 tablespoons reduced-sodium soy sauce

1 tablespoon fresh ginger root, peeled and minced

½ tablespoon garlic, minced

FOR THE SALAD:

2½ cups green cabbage, thinly sliced

1 cup red cabbage, thinly sliced

1 cup Napa cabbage, shredded

1 red bell pepper, thinly sliced

1 carrot, julienned

3 green onions, chopped

¼ cup fresh cilantro, chopped

- Spray a pan with nonstick cooking spray. Grill the chicken 6–8 minutes on each side, remove from heat, and set aside.
- In a medium bowl, whisk together all the salad dressing ingredients. Next, in a large bowl, mix together all the salad ingredients. Add in the chicken. Toss with the peanut butter dressing just before serving.

SERVES 6

The Miracle Carb Diet Nutritional Content for Journaling
Per serving: 0 g carbohydrate, 4 g fiber

Actual Nutritional Content

Per serving: 315 calories, 13 g carbohydrate, 4 g fiber, 32 g protein, 15 g total
 fat, 2 g sat. fat, 547 mg sodium

REBECCA'S HEARTS OF PALM SALAD

*Let's face it, sometimes you're not in the mood for lettuce. That's why F-Factor
dietitian Rebecca came up with this salad as a welcome departure from the
romaine leaves we've grown accustomed to. Hearts of palm make the base of
this easy and delicious dish.*

2 (15-ounce) cans hearts of
 palm, sliced into rings

¼ ripe avocado, cut into small
 cubes

½ container grape or cherry
 tomatoes, halved

¼ cup fresh flat-leaf parsley,
 roughly chopped

Juice of 2 lemons

2 teaspoons salt

1 teaspoon pepper

¼ red onion, finely chopped
 (optional)

½ clove garlic, minced
 (optional)

In a large bowl, add all the ingredients and mix thoroughly. Either serve
right away or set aside for about 30 minutes to enhance flavor.

SERVES 6

The Miracle Carb Diet Nutritional Content for Journaling

Per serving: 0 g carbohydrate, 3 g fiber

Actual Nutritional Content

Per serving: 55 calories, 9 g carbohydrate, 3 g fiber, 3 g protein, 2 g total fat,
 0 g sat. fat, 320 mg sodium

CUCUMBER SALAD

Cucumber Salad is one of my all-time deli favorites. It's cold and refreshing, making it the perfect summer side. I love that this vegetable salad has a slight sweetness to it. Make this dish for your next picnic or backyard barbecue!

2 English cucumbers, thinly sliced

1 small white onion, thinly sliced

2 teaspoons salt, plus more to taste

2 tablespoons white or red wine vinegar

1 tablespoon fresh or 1 teaspoon dried dill, finely chopped

- Toss the cucumbers and onion slices in a large colander with the salt. Place the colander over a bowl to catch draining liquid and refrigerate for 1–2 hours. The cucumbers will shrink considerably as the salt releases their moisture.
- Rinse the cucumbers and onions under cold running water to rinse off the salt, and place on paper towels for about 20 minutes to absorb excess moisture.
- Toss the cucumbers and onion with wine vinegar, dill, and a pinch of salt, if desired. Cover and refrigerate until ready to serve.

SERVES 4

The Miracle Carb Diet Nutritional Content for Journaling
Per serving: 0 g carbohydrate, 2 g fiber

Actual Nutritional Content
Per serving: 45 calories, 9 g carbohydrate, 2 g fiber, 1.5 g protein, 0 g total fat, 0 g sat. fat, 1,173 mg sodium

SOUPS

CREAMY BROCCOLI SOUP

This recipe is simple, delicious, and easy to make. It's thick and flavorful without the addition of fattening cheese or cream. Chock-full of vitamin C and fiber, it packs a one-two nutrition and flavor punch!

1 (12-ounce) microwavable
    steamer bag broccoli
1 carton Mori-Nu Silken Lite
    Firm Tofu
¼ cup grated Parmesan cheese

1 (32-ounce) carton broccoli
    soup (such as Campbell's V8
    or Imagine)
½ tablespoon salt
¼ tablespoon pepper

- Microwave the broccoli steamer bag for 9 minutes until the veggies are extra tender.
- While the broccoli is steaming, place the tofu and Parmesan cheese in either a food processor or blender. Puree the tofu mixture until a cream cheese–like consistency.
- Add the broccoli to the processor and continue to pulse, until totally pureed and thick.
- Add the broccoli soup, along with salt and pepper, to the processor slowly, a little at a time, until all of it has fully blended.
- Pour soup mixture into a pot and heat until simmering. Serve and enjoy!

SERVES 6

The Miracle Carb Diet Nutritional Content for Journaling
Per serving: 0 g carbohydrate, 3 g fiber

Actual Nutritional Content
Per serving: 218 calories, 15 g carbohydrate, 3 g fiber, 13 g protein, 13 g total fat, 5 g sat. fat, 587 mg sodium

CARROT GINGER SOUP

Colorful and fragrant, this is a light soup with just a touch of sweetness. Carrots are packed with beta-carotene, which is important for eye health, and ginger is a good source of antioxidants. Plus, the combination of the two just tastes great!

Nonstick cooking spray

2 shallots, minced

4 tablespoons fresh ginger, peeled and minced

2 pounds carrots, peeled and chopped

4 cups reduced sodium vegetable or chicken broth

2 cups water

½ teaspoon coriander or fresh cilantro

Pinch ground cinnamon

1 teaspoon salt

Snipped fresh chives or parsley, for garnish

- Heat a pot over medium-high heat, and spray with nonstick cooking spray.
- Add the shallots and sauté until tender, about 5 minutes. Add the ginger and sauté for another 3–4 minutes.
- Add the carrots, broth, water, coriander or cilantro, cinnamon, and salt, and bring to a boil.
- Reduce heat to a simmer and cook for 10–15 minutes, or until carrots are tender. Carefully transfer to a blender and puree.
- Pour soup mixture back into the pot and heat until warmed through. Garnish with chives or parsley to serve.

SERVES 12

The Miracle Carb Diet Nutritional Content for Journaling
Per serving: 0 g carbohydrate, 14 g fiber

Actual Nutritional Content
Per serving: 268 calories, 58 g carbohydrate, 14 g fiber, 10 g protein, 2 g total fat, 0 g sat. fat, 980 mg sodium

FRENCH ONION SOUP

French Onion Soup is one of the most popular soups there is, and luckily it's one of the easiest to prepare. The rich broth is complemented perfectly by the sweetness of the caramelized onions and the sharpness of the cheese. Enjoy a bowlful of this classic favorite.

1 tablespoon olive oil

10 medium onions, thinly sliced

1 tablespoon water

1 teaspoon dried thyme

¼ teaspoon pepper

¼ cup port wine or sherry

5 cups low-sodium vegetable broth

2 tablespoons balsamic vinegar

6 tablespoons grated Parmesan cheese

6 high-fiber crackers, to serve

- Preheat the oven to 450 °F.
- In a large Dutch oven, add the olive oil, onions, water, thyme, and pepper. Cover and bake for 30 minutes, until the onions are soft and start to turn brown.
- Uncover and continue to bake for another 30 minutes or so, until the onions are golden brown and caramelized.
- Transfer the Dutch oven to the stove and turn burner to medium heat. Add the wine, and scrape the bottom and sides of the pan to release any browned parts.
- Continue to cook until mixture is slightly thickened. Add the broth and vinegar. Bring to a boil, then reduce heat and simmer for about 15 minutes, until the liquid has darkened.
- Divide soup into bowls, add 1 tablespoon of Parmesan cheese to each bowl, and top with a high-fiber cracker. Serve immediately.

SERVES 6

The Miracle Carb Diet Nutritional Content for Journaling
Per serving: 4 g carbohydrate, 8 g fiber

Actual Nutritional Content

Per serving: 63 calories, 4 g carbohydrate, 1 g fiber, 3 g protein, 2 g total fat, 0 g sat. fat, 2,728 mg sodium

SHREDDED CABBAGE SOUP

Many of us may recall the Cabbage Soup Diet. You could eat all the cabbage soup you wanted and you lost weight. The reason? Cabbage soup is low in calories. Another bonus? Cabbage is loaded with cancer-fighting antioxidants. So fill up!

Nonstick cooking spray

3 cloves garlic, finely chopped

1 medium onion, finely chopped

4 carrots, peeled and cut into 1-inch chunks

3 stalks celery, cut into 1-inch slices

4 cups beef stock

1 pound (about ½ head) Napa cabbage, shredded

2 cups crushed canned tomatoes

6 tablespoons (about 1½ lemons) lemon juice

2 tablespoons fresh dill, chopped

½ teaspoon fresh thyme

1 tablespoon salt

½ tablespoon pepper

- Place a pot over medium-high heat and spray with nonstick cooking spray. Add the garlic, onion, carrots, celery, and ½ cup beef stock, and cook for about 5 minutes.
- Add the cabbage and the remaining beef stock, and simmer for 15 minutes.
- Add the tomatoes, lemon juice, dill, thyme, salt, and pepper, and simmer for 20 minutes.

SERVES 8 (1 CUP PER SERVING)

The Miracle Carb Diet Nutritional Content for Journaling

Per serving: 0 g carbohydrate, 4 g fiber

Actual Nutritional Content

Per serving: 177 calories, 18 g carbohydrate, 4 g fiber, 11 g protein, 7 g total
fat, 3 g sat. fat, 1,011 mg sodium

THAI CHICKEN COCONUT SOUP

*This quick and easy soup is filled with distinctive flavors, such as coconut,
ginger, and lime. This is a delicious twist on a traditional and tasty Thai favorite. The soup is mild, creamy, and rich, and sure to tantalize your taste buds.*

¼ cup fresh ginger, peeled and grated

2 cloves garlic, chopped

1 chili pepper, sliced

4 cups reduced-sodium chicken broth

½ pound boneless, skinless chicken tenders

½ cup light coconut milk

2 tablespoons cornstarch

1 tablespoon lemon juice

2 tablespoons lime juice

1 tablespoon fish sauce

¼ cup scallions, sliced

- In a large pan over medium-high heat, add the ginger, garlic, chili pepper, and chicken broth. Bring to a boil, then reduce heat to a simmer.
- Add the chicken tenders to the broth. Cover and simmer gently over a
low heat until the chicken is cooked through, about 5–7 minutes. Stir
in the coconut milk.
- In a small bowl, whisk together the cornstarch, lemon juice, lime juice,
and fish sauce. Add the cornstarch mixture to the broth, and simmer
over medium heat until the soup has thickened slightly.
- Right before serving, sprinkle with scallions.

SERVES 8

The Miracle Carb Diet Nutritional Content for Journaling

Per serving: 2 g carbohydrate, .5 g fiber

Actual Nutritional Content

Per serving: 114 calories, 6 g carbohydrate, .5 g fiber, 7 g protein, 5 g total
fat, 4 g sat. fat, 261 mg sodium

POULTRY

SOUTHERN "FRIED" CHICKEN

Yes, you read correctly. This is a recipe for delicious crispy chicken. See, I told you that healthy food doesn't have to be boring! The crunchy coating on this chicken seals in the juices, giving this southern standard its finger-licking flavor without the extra calories.

Nonstick cooking spray

¾ cup fat-free buttermilk

3 pounds boneless, skinless
   chicken tenders

½ cup cracker crumbs (3 high-
   fiber crackers, crushed)

1½ teaspoons paprika

1½ teaspoons salt

½ teaspoon pepper

- Preheat the oven to 400 °F. Coat a baking pan with nonstick cooking spray. Set aside.
- Pour the buttermilk into a shallow bowl. Add the chicken, turning to coat. Refrigerate for at least 15 minutes, turning occasionally. In another shallow dish, combine the cracker crumbs with the paprika, salt, and pepper.
- One at a time, dip each side of the chicken into the cracker mixture, pressing firmly to coat. Place on the prepared baking pan.
- Coat the chicken with nonstick spray. Bake for ten minutes, then turn the pieces over and continue to bake for 10 minutes more, until the chicken is crisp and golden brown.

Tip: If you cannot find nonfat buttermilk at your market, you can substitute 1 cup of nonfat Greek yogurt, thinned out with 3 tablespoons of water.

SERVES 12

The Miracle Carb Diet Nutritional Content for Journaling
Per serving: 10 g carbohydrate, 7.5 g fiber

Actual Nutritional Content
Per serving: 154 calories, 3 g carbohydrate, 1 g fiber, 28 g protein, 3 g total fat, 1 g sat. fat, 575 mg sodium

TURKEY MEATBALLS

Spaghetti and meatballs has always been a family favorite, so it's no wonder that this dish is most parents' go-to meal. However, an average serving of four meatballs can have as much as 560 calories and 42 grams of fat. By swapping traditional meats for fat-free ground turkey breast, you can drastically reduce both the calorie and fat content and give your family a meal you'll feel good to serve.

Nonstick cooking spray
½ pound ground turkey breast
1 cup cracker crumbs (6 high-fiber crackers, crushed)
8 scallions, finely diced
½ cup (about 6 large) button mushrooms, chopped

1 small onion, diced
2 egg whites, plus 1 egg
2–3 cloves garlic, peeled and minced
1 tablespoon salt
½ tablespoon pepper
½ cup tomato sauce (optional)

- Preheat the oven to 350 °F. Lightly coat a 4 × 8-inch loaf pan with nonstick cooking spray.
- In a large bowl, add the turkey, cracker crumbs, scallions, mushrooms,

onion, egg whites, egg, garlic, salt, and pepper in a bowl. Mix until thoroughly combined.

- Roll the mixture into twelve meatballs and place on the prepared pan.
- Bake for 30 minutes, or until cooked through and the meatballs have browned. Add tomato sauce to these meatballs, if desired, for pasta or as a side dish, or enjoy plain.

    SERVES 6

The Miracle Carb Diet Nutritional Content for Journaling
Per serving: 24 g carbohydrate, 21 g fiber

Actual Nutritional Content
Per serving: 100 calories, 12 g carbohydrate, 6 g fiber, 11 g protein, 4 g total fat, 1 g sat. fat, 626 mg sodium

HERB ROASTED TURKEY BREAST

Herbs are a great way to add flavor to dishes without adding calories. This Herb Roasted Turkey Breast is juicy, tender, and easy to make. After dinner, you can shred the leftover turkey and use it in salads, soups, and sandwiches. Talk about versatility!

1 (4-pound) fresh bone-in turkey breast, rinsed and patted dry

2 tablespoons olive oil

1 tablespoon garlic, minced

1 tablespoon fresh rosemary leaves, chopped

1 tablespoon fresh sage leaves, chopped

1 teaspoon fresh thyme leaves, chopped

2 teaspoons salt

1 teaspoon pepper

- Preheat the oven to 325 °F.
- Rub the turkey all over with the olive oil.

- Mix the remaining ingredients in a bowl. Season the turkey generously with the herbs.
- Set the turkey in a roasting pan, breast side up, and roast for 2–2½ hours, or until an instant-read thermometer inserted into the thickest part of the roast registers 160 °F.
- Transfer the turkey to a cutting board and let rest for 30 minutes before slicing.

SERVES 12

The Miracle Carb Diet Nutritional Content for Journaling
Per serving: 0 g carbohydrate, 1 g fiber

Actual Nutritional Content
Per serving: 210 calories, 8 g carbohydrate, 1 g fiber, 29 g protein, 6 g total fat, 1 g sat. fat, 2,308 mg sodium

BAKED APRICOT CHICKEN

My kids love this dish because it's something sweet and crunchy for dinner, and I love it because it's actually good for them. You can even swap out the chicken breasts with chicken fingers for the perfect low-calorie party appetizer!

4 (4-ounce) skinless, boneless chicken breasts
½ cup sugar-free apricot preserves (such as Polaner Sugar Free Preserves with Fiber)
½ cup cracker crumbs (3 high-fiber crackers, crushed)

1 teaspoon garlic powder
¼ teaspoon ground ginger
½ teaspoon salt
½ teaspoon pepper

- Preheat the oven to 350 °F.
- Arrange the chicken breasts in a nonstick baking dish. Spread the preserves over the chicken on both sides.
- In a bowl, combine the remaining ingredients. Spread the crumb mixture over both sides of each chicken breast.
- Bake for 20 minutes, or until cooked through.

SERVES 4

The Miracle Carb Diet Nutritional Content for Journaling
Per serving: 5 g carbohydrate, 4 g fiber

Actual Nutritional Content
Per serving: 174 calories, 16 g carbohydrate, 4 g fiber, 28 g protein, 3 g total fat, 1 g sat. fat, 914 mg sodium

CHICKEN CURRY

This dish doesn't take a top chef to prepare; it just tastes like it does! Chicken curry is actually quite simple to make and is a great new answer to the eternal question, "What's for dinner?"

1 pound precooked chicken breast, cut into bite-size pieces

½ pound fresh mushrooms, thinly sliced

1 small onion, chopped

2 tablespoons acceptable vegetable oil or marinade

1 cup homemade chicken broth or commercial low-sodium variety

1½ teaspoons curry powder

½ teaspoon cumin

½ teaspoon turmeric

1 cup apple, finely chopped

¼ cup parsley, chopped

¾ cup light coconut milk

1 cup water

- In a large skillet over medium-high heat, sauté the chicken, mushrooms, and onion in vegetable oil until chicken is lightly browned on all sides.
- Stir in the broth, curry powder, cumin, and turmeric. Next, add the apple and parsley. Pour in the coconut milk and water.
- Simmer, stirring often, for 20 minutes, or until apple pieces are tender but still crisp.

SERVES 4

The Miracle Carb Diet Nutritional Content for Journaling
Per serving: 11 g carbohydrate, 1.5 g fiber

Actual Nutritional Content
Per serving: 185 calories, 11 g carbohydrate, 2 g fiber, 19 g protein, 8 g total fat, 1 g sat. fat, 216 mg sodium

BEEF/PORK/LAMB/VEAL

LAMB CHOPS

There's nothing quite like a succulent, juicy, and tender lamb chop. This is an extremely easy yet elegant dinner that you can get on the table in 30 minutes flat. It makes for the perfect mouth-watering chops every time.

¼ cup Dijon mustard
1 tablespoon parsley, chopped, plus sprigs for garnish
½ teaspoon lemon pepper
1 shallot, chopped

1 clove garlic, chopped
4 (½-pound, 1-inch-thick) lamb chops
Tomato wedges, for garnish
Parsley sprigs, for garnish

- Preheat the broiler.
- In a small bowl, combine the mustard, parsley, lemon pepper, shallot, and garlic.
- On a broiler pan, arrange the lamb chops. Spread half the mustard

mixture over the chops. Broil 5–6 inches from the heat source, about 6–7 minutes, or until browned.

- Turn the chops, and spread the remaining mustard mixture evenly over them. Broil 6–7 minutes, or until browned. Garnish with the tomato wedges and parsley sprigs to serve.

SERVES 4

The Miracle Carb Diet Nutritional Content for Journaling
Per serving: 0 g carbohydrate, 0 g fiber

Actual Nutritional Content
Per serving: 363 calories, 4.5 g carbohydrate, 0 g fiber, 47 g protein, 16 g total fat, 5 g sat. fat, 263 mg sodium

GARLIC-CHILI FLANK STEAK

Ladies and gentlemen, red meat is not off the menu. This steak is succulent and tender, and the garlic-chili spice rub gives it just the right amount of heat. My husband swears by this steak, and I think you will, too.

2 cloves garlic, minced	1 teaspoon dried oregano
¼ cup white vinegar	1 teaspoon ground cumin
2 teaspoons olive oil	¼ teaspoon salt
2 teaspoons ground ancho chili pepper	1 pound flank steak, trimmed of fat

- Whisk the garlic, vinegar, olive oil, ground chili, oregano, cumin, and salt in a small bowl. Place the steak in a shallow baking dish and pour the marinade over it, turning to coat both sides.
- Cover and refrigerate for at least 30 minutes, turning once.
- Preheat the grill to high heat or preheat the broiler. Grill the steak until desired doneness, 5–6 minutes per side for medium (or, if broiling in the oven, cook for about 8 minutes per side).
- Transfer to a plate, cover with foil, and let rest for 5 minutes.

- Slice the steak very thinly across the grain. Serve warm or chilled.

SERVES 4 (4 OUNCES PER SERVING)

The Miracle Carb Diet Nutritional Content for Journaling
Per serving: 0 g carbohydrate, 1 g fiber

Actual Nutritional Content
Per serving: 237 calories, 0 g carbohydrate, 1 g fiber, 24 g protein, 17 g fat, 6 g sat. fat, 192 mg sodium

FILET MIGNON WITH CREAMY HORSERADISH SAUCE

Filet mignon goes bold with the addition of horseradish sauce. The horseradish adds a delicious kick to the juicy beef that makes this dish anything but average. Keep your portion about the size of a deck of cards. Steak's on!

Nonstick cooking spray
1 (3½-pound) center-cut beef tenderloin, trimmed and cut into filets
2 teaspoons olive oil

1 teaspoon garlic powder
1 teaspoon onion powder
½ tablespoon salt
2 teaspoons pepper

FOR THE HORSERADISH SAUCE:

1 cup fat-free mayonnaise
1 cup fat-free Greek yogurt
1 tablespoon Dijon-style mustard

2 green onions, finely chopped
¼ cup prepared horseradish
1 teaspoon white wine vinegar

- Preheat the oven to 400 °F. Spray a large, heavy roasting pan with nonstick cooking spray.
- Place the tenderloin in the pan. Rub the tenderloin with the olive oil, and season lightly on all sides with the garlic powder, onion powder, salt, and pepper.

- Place the roasting pan on the stovetop over medium-high heat, and sear the meat on all sides, about 5–6 minutes per side. Place in the oven for about 20–25 minutes for medium-rare.
- Meanwhile, in a bowl, combine all the horseradish sauce ingredients and blend well. Refrigerate until ready to serve.

SERVES 12

The Miracle Carb Diet Nutritional Content for Journaling
Per serving: 0 g carbohydrate, 0 g fiber

Actual Nutritional Content
Per serving: 276 calories, 4 g carbohydrate, 0 g fiber, 41 g protein, 14 g total fat, 5 g sat. fat, 243 mg sodium

PORK CHOPS WITH APPLES AND ONIONS

It's hard to resist this classic combination, and now you don't have to! Many people assume that pork is a fatty meat, but pork chops can actually be a relatively lean cut. In this dish, the savory chop is complemented perfectly by the sweet, spiced apples and savory onions.

4 (4-ounce) lean boneless pork loin chops

½ teaspoon salt

¼–½ teaspoon pepper

Nonstick cooking spray

⅓ cup reduced-sodium chicken stock

1 cup onion, sliced

2 large gala or golden delicious apples, peeled and chopped

1 packet nonnutritive sweetener

3 tablespoons red wine vinegar

6 sprigs fresh thyme, leaves finely chopped

- Season the pork chops with salt and pepper. Spray a medium skillet with nonstick cooking spray and place over medium-high heat.
- Cook the chops until golden, 3–4 minutes per side. Remove the cooked chops to a plate and cover to keep warm.

- Add the remaining ingredients to the skillet. Stir the sauce over medium-high heat until the apples are soft, about 10 minutes. Add the pork chops back to the skillet and cook for 10 more minutes, turning once at about 5 minutes, until pork chops are cooked through.

SERVES 4

The Miracle Carb Diet Nutritional Content for Journaling
Per serving: 10 g carbohydrate, 3 g fiber

Actual Nutritional Content
Per serving: 208 calories, 18 g carbohydrate, 3 g fiber, 26 g protein, 4 g total fat, 1 g sat. fat, 562 mg sodium

VEAL MARSALA

This recipe tops tender veal scallops with a light mushroom Marsala wine sauce. It's a great dinner for any night of the week, as it is quick, easy, and delicious. Be sure to use dry Marsala wine so that your sauce doesn't come out too sweet!

6 (4-ounce) veal cutlets
1 teaspoon salt
2 teaspoons pepper
¼ teaspoon dried oregano
¼ teaspoon dried thyme
Nonstick cooking spray
1 large shallot, finely chopped
3 cloves garlic, smashed

2 tablespoons fresh Italian parsley, chopped
2 ounces (about 10–15) cremini mushrooms
½ cup dry Marsala wine
1 cup chicken broth
1 tablespoon lemon juice

- Sprinkle the veal with salt, pepper, oregano, and thyme.
- Spray a large skillet with nonstick cooking spray and put over medium-high heat.

- Working in batches, add three veal cutlets at a time to the skillet and cook until golden brown, about 1½ minutes per side. Transfer the veal to a plate. Spray the skillet again if necessary. Repeat with the remaining three cutlets. Set the cutlets aside.
- Spray the skillet with nonstick cooking spray, if needed, and add the shallot, garlic, and parsley. Sauté until fragrant, about 30 seconds.
- Add the mushrooms and cook about 3 minutes, until tender and the juices evaporate. Add the Marsala wine and simmer about 2 minutes. Add the broth and lemon juice and simmer about 4 minutes, or until the sauce has reduced by half.
- Put the veal cutlets back into the skillet and cook cutlets so they are heated through.

SERVES 6

The Miracle Carb Diet Nutritional Content for Journaling
Per serving: 3 g carbohydrate, 0 g fiber

Actual Nutritional Content
Per serving: 196 calories, 4 g carbohydrate, 0 g fiber, 24 g protein, 6 g total fat, 3 g sat. fat, 490 mg sodium

FISH/SEAFOOD

STEAMED "MISO-GLAZED" COD

This is an extremely popular dish served up in Japanese restaurants. In this entrée, delectably buttery cod meets its perfect match with a sweet miso glaze. Cod is a white meat fish that becomes incredibly moist when cooked due to its high healthy fat content. Who knew steamed fish could taste so good?

½ cup light miso paste

¼ cup rice vinegar

1 tablespoon nonnutritive
sweetener

2 tablespoons soy sauce

¼ teaspoon cayenne pepper

2 tablespoons olive oil

1 pound white cod fillet

2 tablespoons fresh cilantro,
chopped, for garnish

- Preheat the oven to 450 °F.
- Blend the miso, vinegar, nonnutritive sweetener, soy sauce, and cayenne pepper in a food processor. With the machine running, gradually pour in the olive oil, blending until mixture is smooth. (You can also whisk it by hand.)
- Place the cod fillet on a baking sheet lined with parchment paper. Pour the miso sauce over the cod on all sides. Cover and refrigerate for about 15 minutes.
- Broil the cod until the miso glaze starts to brown, about 3–5 minutes. Transfer from the broiler to the middle of the oven and bake until the fish is opaque in the center, about another 20–25 minutes. Sprinkle with fresh cilantro and serve immediately.

SERVES 4

The Miracle Carb Diet Nutritional Content for Journaling
Per serving: 0 g carbohydrate, 2.5 g fiber

Actual Nutritional Content
Per serving: 240 calories, 10 g carbohydrate, 2.5 g fiber, 26 g protein, 10 g total fat, 1.5 g sat. fat, 1,618 mg sodium

MUSSELS WITH A QUICK TOMATO SAUCE

Mussels marinara is an easy and affordable, yet elegant dish. The mussels are simply steamed in a fragrant tomato broth. Once the mussels open up, it's time to pour a glass of wine and enjoy!

1 tablespoon olive oil

1 small onion, diced

2 cloves garlic, chopped

12 plum tomatoes,
   chopped

8 basil leaves

2 teaspoons salt

½ tablespoon pepper

½ cup white wine

4 pounds mussels, cleaned and
   debearded

2 tablespoons fresh parsley,
   chopped

- Heat the olive oil in a large saucepot over medium heat. Add the onion and garlic, and sauté until translucent, about 2 minutes. Add the chopped tomatoes, basil, salt, pepper, and white wine, and cook for about 10 minutes.
- Next, add the mussels to the pot and cover with a lid and let simmer until the mussels have opened up, about 10 minutes. Discard any mussels that do not open. Sprinkle with freshly chopped parsley.

SERVES 6

The Miracle Carb Diet Nutritional Content for Journaling
Per serving: 0 g carbohydrate, 3 g fiber

Actual Nutritional Content
Per serving: 210 calories, 15 g carbohydrate, 3 g fiber, 19.5 g protein, 6 g total fat, 1 g sat. fat, 1,655 mg sodium

SWEET MANGO SALMON

Give your standard salmon fillet a surprisingly sweet twist. Mango salsa not only adds a delicious burst of flavor but also a beautiful burst of color. This dish looks great, tastes great, and packs essential nutrients that will help you feel great, too!

Nonstick cooking spray

4 (4-ounce) salmon fish
fillets

6 pieces dried unsweetened
mango, chopped

3 tablespoons mustard

1 tablespoon orange juice

¼ cup light soy sauce

1 tablespoon fresh lemon juice

1 teaspoon olive oil

1 packet nonnutritive
sweetener

½ teaspoon salt

½ teaspoon pepper

½ teaspoon garlic powder

½ teaspoon onion powder

- Preheat the oven to 400 °F. Lightly spray a baking dish with nonstick cooking spray.
- Place the salmon and mango in the baking dish.
- In a bowl, combine the mustard, orange juice, soy sauce, lemon juice, and olive oil. Whisk together until fully combined. Add the rest of the ingredients to the sauce and stir.
- Pour the sauce over the salmon and mango.
- Bake for 20–25 minutes, or until the salmon is cooked through.

SERVES 4

The Miracle Carb Diet Nutritional Content for Journaling
Per serving: 6 g carbohydrate, 1 g fiber

Actual Nutritional Content
Per serving: 216 calories, 10 g carbohydrate, 1 g fiber, 24 g protein, 9 g total fat, 1 g sat. fat, 1,000 mg sodium

SESAME-CRUSTED SEARED TUNA

This is a beautiful and simple way to serve one of the tastiest fish around. The tuna is coated with sesame seeds and quickly seared. I like to serve this dish rare, so be sure to get high-quality fresh tuna steaks.

1 cup low-sodium soy sauce

2 tablespoons green onion, finely chopped

2 packets nonnutritive sweetener

4 (4-ounce) tuna fillets

Nonstick cooking spray

8 tablespoons toasted sesame seeds

- In a small bowl, combine the soy sauce, green onion, and nonnutritive sweetener, mixing well.
- Place the tuna in glass baking dish and pour the marinade over it. Marinate for at least 15 minutes.
- Coat a cast-iron or heavy-bottomed skillet with nonstick cooking spray, and heat over medium-high heat.
- Coat the tuna fillets on all sides with sesame seeds. Cook each tuna fillet for 3–5 minutes on each side, or to desired doneness.

SERVES 4

The Miracle Carb Diet Nutritional Content for Journaling
Per serving: 0 g carbohydrate, 4 g fiber

Actual Nutritional Content
Per serving: 265 calories, 11 g carbohydrate, 4 g fiber, 33 g protein, 10 g total fat, 2 g sat. fat, 2,174 mg sodium

SPICY CREOLE SHRIMP

This Gulf Coast classic might just get you dreaming of the bayou. Shrimp is one of my favorite proteins to cook with, because it's low in calories and is ready in a snap. The complex spicy flavors will only make it look like you spent hours in the kitchen.

Nonstick cooking spray

3 cloves garlic, minced

24 medium shrimp, peeled and deveined

¼ cup Tabasco Sauce

½ cup white wine

¼ cup fresh parsley, chopped

- Spray a large skillet with nonstick cooking spray, and heat over medium-high heat. Add the garlic to the skillet, and cook for 1 minute. Add the shrimp to the skillet, and sauté with the garlic for 1 minute.
- Add the remaining ingredients, and let the shrimp simmer in the sauce until the shrimp are cooked through, about 5–7 minutes. Serve hot.

    SERVES 6

The Miracle Carb Diet Nutritional Content for Journaling
Per serving: 0 g carbohydrate, 0 g fiber

Actual Nutritional Content
Per serving: 53 calories, 1 g carbohydrate, 0 g fiber, 7 g protein, 0 g fat, 0 g sat. fat, 104 mg sodium

SIDES

ZUCCHINI "CARPACCIO"

Carpaccio is an Italian delicacy of thinly sliced raw meat or fish. However, this recipe is a vegetarian version of carpaccio, and it's surprisingly quick and easy to make.

4 tablespoons olive oil

2 tablespoons (about ½ lemon) fresh lemon juice

2 medium zucchini, ends cut off and thinly sliced

1 teaspoon salt

1 teaspoon pepper

1 cup baby arugula

¼ cup reduced-fat Parmesan cheese, thinly shaved

- Whisk together the oil and lemon juice in a small bowl.
- In a large platter or dish, place a layer of zucchini to cover the bottom of the platter. Sprinkle with salt and pepper, and drizzle with the mixture of olive oil and lemon juice. Repeat, layering the zucchini, salt, pepper, and olive oil–lemon juice mixture, until all the zucchini is used up.

- Let marinate for at least 10 minutes. Right before serving, top with fresh arugula and shaved Parmesan.

    SERVES 4

The Miracle Carb Diet Nutritional Content for Journaling
Per serving: 0 g carbohydrate, 1 g fiber

Actual Nutritional Content
Per serving: 86 calories, 7 g carbohydrate, 1 g fiber, 4 g protein, 5 g total fat,
    1 g sat. fat, 98 mg sodium

BLACKENED BROCCOLI

When my assistant, Jessica, found out I was writing a book, she begged for me to include her burnt broccoli recipe. I wasn't exactly thrilled with the idea of including recipes where the food was "burnt" until I tried her amazing side dish. Kudos, Jess.

Nonstick cooking spray	1 tablespoon garlic, minced
1 head broccoli	¼ teaspoon salt
1 tablespoon olive oil	⅛ teaspoon pepper
1 teaspoon lemon juice	1 tablespoon balsamic vinegar

- Preheat the oven to 400 °F. Line a baking sheet with tinfoil, and spray with nonstick cooking spray.
- Cut off the broccoli stems and discard. Cut remaining broccoli into bite-size florets.
- In a large plastic Ziploc bag, place the broccoli and the remaining ingredients, seal the bag, and shake, until the broccoli is evenly coated (feel free to allow the broccoli to marinate for 10–20 minutes).
- Spread the broccoli pieces onto the prepared baking sheet.
- Bake the broccoli for 40 minutes, or until the broccoli is slightly blackened and crispy.

    SERVES 4

The Miracle Carb Diet Nutritional Content for Journaling
Per serving: 0 g carbohydrate, 4 g fiber

Actual Nutritional Content
Per serving: 89 calories, 12 g carbohydrate, 4 g fiber, 4 g protein, 4 g total
fat, .5 g sat. fat, 197 mg sodium

OVEN-"FRIED" ARTICHOKE HEARTS

Whenever our F-Factor team has something to celebrate, we head straight to Cipriani. Our favorite dish there? Crispy artichokes. Artichokes are one of the highest-fiber vegetables out there, and this addictive recipe makes them melt-in-your-mouth good. They are definitely something to celebrate.

Nonstick cooking spray

3 (9-ounce) boxes Birds Eye
   Artichoke Hearts, thawed

1 tablespoon onion salt

½ tablespoon pepper

- Preheat the oven to 400 °F. Coat a baking dish with nonstick cooking spray.
- Add the artichoke hearts to the baking dish.
- Add the onion salt and pepper, and mix until the artichoke hearts are evenly coated with seasonings. Lightly spray nonstick cooking spray on the artichoke hearts.
- Bake the artichoke until edges are golden brown, about 35–40 minutes.

SERVES 8

The Miracle Carb Diet Nutritional Content for Journaling
Per serving: 0 g carbohydrate, 6 g fiber

Actual Nutritional Content
Per serving: 60 calories, 9 g carbohydrate, 6 g fiber, 2 g protein, 2 g total fat,
1 g sat. fat, 53 mg sodium

STUFFED MUSHROOMS

It's time to give mushrooms the spotlight. Believe it or not, 1 cup of mushrooms has just 20 calories, 3 grams of carbohydrate, and 0 grams of fat. Try this recipe with some protein for a meal, or eat it on its own as an appetizer or snack.

Nonstick cooking spray

4 fresh portabella mushrooms

1 (10-ounce) package of spinach, thawed and squeezed dry with a paper towel

1 small onion, chopped

1 cup low-fat ricotta cheese

¼ cup grated Parmesan cheese

¼ cup cracker crumbs (1½ high-fiber crackers, crushed)

¼ cup marinara sauce

- Preheat the oven to 400 °F. Spray a baking sheet with nonstick cooking spray.
- Clean the mushrooms and remove the stems. Arrange the mushroom caps on the prepared baking sheet. Set aside.
- Spray a sauté pan with nonstick cooking spray and set over medium heat. Add the spinach and onion, then sauté until the onions are soft and translucent. Transfer to a small bowl.
- Combine the sautéed spinach and onion with the ricotta cheese. In another small bowl, mix the Parmesan cheese and cracker crumbs together.
- Using a spoon, fill each mushroom cap with a generous amount of the spinach mixture.
- Spoon the marinara sauce over the mushrooms, and sprinkle with the cheese-cracker topping. Bake in the oven for 15 minutes, or until golden.

SERVES 4

The Miracle Carb Diet Nutritional Content for Journaling
Per serving: 3 g carbohydrate, 6 g fiber

Actual Nutritional Content

Per serving: 166 calories, 16 g carbohydrate, 6 g fiber, 14 g protein, 7 g total
    fat, 4 g sat. fat, 412 mg sodium

BRUSSELS SPROUTS

*Brussels sprouts are often coated in a sweet honey glaze or sautéed in bacon
grease to make them more than the everyday fare. Both of these cooking
methods add unnecessary calories to an otherwise healthy side dish. In order to steer away from these high-calorie additions, I season the Brussels
sprouts with a mixture of Asian spices (star anise, cinnamon, cloves) and a
touch of soy sauce.*

1 pound Brussels sprouts

Nonstick cooking spray

3 scallions, sliced

1 teaspoon fresh ginger, peeled
    and shredded

2 cloves garlic, minced

1/8 teaspoon ground cinnamon

1/8 teaspoon ground star anise

Pinch ground cloves

1 teaspoon pepper

1 tablespoon low-sodium soy
    sauce

- Trim the stem ends of the Brussels sprouts. Then slice the Brussels
  sprouts with a large, sharp knife (they will appear as if you had shredded them).
- Spray a large nonstick skillet with nonstick cooking spray, and heat
  over medium heat. Add the scallions, ginger, and garlic, and sauté for
  about 1 minute.
- Add the Brussels sprouts, spices, and soy sauce, and continue to cook
  for another 5–7 minutes, or until the Brussels sprouts are tender.

    SERVES 4

The Miracle Carb Diet Nutritional Content for Journaling

Per serving: 7 g carbohydrate, 5 g fiber

Actual Nutritional Content

Per serving: 60 calories, 12 g carbohydrate, 5 g fiber, 4 g protein, 0 g total fat, 0 g sat. fat, 164 mg sodium

DESSERTS

COCOA PEANUT BUTTER FLYING SAUCER

Growing up, my mother always kept a package of ice cream sandwiches in the freezer. They were my favorite after-dinner treat, and with my healthy take on this dessert, I can now enjoy them anytime. I've made a sweet and creamy peanut butter spread to sandwich between two high-fiber crackers.

1 6 oz. container fat-free Greek yogurt

2 tablespoons nonnutritive sweetener

6 tablespoons PB2

½ tablespoon unsweetened cocoa powder

2 high-fiber crackers

- In a large bowl, add the yogurt, nonnutritive sweetener, PB2, and cocoa powder. Use a handheld mixer or mix by hand, blending the peanut butter mixture until smooth.
- Spoon mixture onto one of the high-fiber crackers and top with the other cracker.

SERVES 2

The Miracle Carb Diet Nutritional Content for Journaling

Per serving: 9 g carbohydrate, 8 g fiber

Actual Nutritional Content

Per serving: 137 calories, 20 g carbohydrate, 8 g fiber, 19 g protein, 2 g total fat, 0 g sat. fat, 173 mg sodium

MAKE YOUR OWN POPSICLES
(THREE DIFFERENT WAYS)

Kids (and adults) love anything sweet on a stick. These cool, refreshing treats are a cinch to make, and you will love these popsicles to the last lick!

CRAN-POM POPSICLE

½ cup orange juice

½ cup cranberry-pomegranate juice

10 mint leaves, thinly sliced

SPECIAL EQUIPMENT:

Dixie 2-Ounce Portion Cups

Popsicle sticks

- Mix the orange juice, cranberry-pomegranate juice, and mint in a small bowl.
- Pour equal amounts of mixture into four Dixie cups.
- Add a popsicle stick to each cup and freeze.

   SERVES 4

The Miracle Carb Diet Nutritional Content for Journaling
Per serving: 8 g carbohydrate, 0 g fiber

Actual Nutritional Content
Per serving: 33 calories, 8 g carbohydrate, 0 g fiber, 0 g protein, 0 g fat, 0 g sat. fat, 1 mg sodium

LEMONADE POPSICLE

1 cup Vitaminwater Zero Squeezed (lemonade flavor)

5 mint leaves, thinly sliced

5 basil leaves, thinly sliced

Dixie 2-Ounce Portion Cups   Popsicle sticks

- Mix all the ingredients in a small bowl.
- Pour equal amounts of mixture into four Dixie cups.
- Add a Popsicle stick to each cup and freeze.

SERVES 4

The Miracle Carb Diet Nutritional Content for Journaling

Per serving: 1 g carbohydrate, 0 g fiber

Actual Nutritional Content

Per serving: 13 calories, 1 g carbohydrate, 0 g fiber, 0 g protein, 0 g fat, 0 g sat. fat, 0 mg sodium

PINEAPPLE-BLUEBERRY-RASPBERRY POPSICLE

1 cup pineapple juice   12 raspberries, washed
12 blueberries, washed

SPECIAL EQUIPMENT:
Dixie 2-Ounce Portion Cups   Popsicle sticks

- Pour equal amounts of pineapple juice into four Dixie cups.
- Drop 3 blueberries and 3 raspberries into each cup.
- Add a Popsicle stick to each cup and freeze.

SERVES 4

The Miracle Carb Diet Nutritional Content for Journaling

Per serving: 9 g carbohydrate, 3 g fiber

Actual Nutritional Content

Per serving: 38 calories, 9 g carbohydrate, 3 g fiber, 0 g protein, 0 g fat, 0 g sat. fat, 0 mg sodium

PEACH CRISP WITH
SWEET VANILLA SAUCE

There's nothing like digging your fork into a warm dessert fresh from the oven. This dessert tastes decadent but is surprisingly low in calories and fat. The vanilla sauce adds a hint of sweetness to the cinnamon crumble, making this dessert an absolute standout.

Nonstick cooking spray

1 cup frozen sliced peaches, thawed

1–2 packets nonnutritive sweetener

1 tablespoon lemon juice

¼ cup Kellogg's All-Bran Bran Buds cereal, crushed

½ teaspoon cinnamon

FOR THE SWEET VANILLA SAUCE:

½ cup Greek yogurt

¼ teaspoon cinnamon

¼ teaspoon vanilla extract

- Preheat the oven to 375 °F. Coat an 8 × 8-inch baking dish with nonstick cooking spray.
- Combine the peaches, nonnutritive sweetener, and lemon juice in a large bowl. Place the peach mixture into the prepared baking dish.
- In a small bowl, combine the Bran Buds and cinnamon. Sprinkle mixture on top of the peaches.
- Cover with foil and bake for 25 minutes. Meanwhile, combine all the ingredients for the vanilla sauce (adding just enough water to thin out to a sauce consistency).
- Serve with the peach crisp on the side or drizzled on top.

SERVES 4

The Miracle Carb Diet Nutritional Content for Journaling
Per serving: 9 g carbohydrate, 4 g fiber

Actual Nutritional Content

Per serving: 70 calories, 17 g carbohydrate, 4 g fiber, 0 g protein, 0 g total fat, 0 g sat. fat, 4 mg sodium

CHEESECAKE

Cheesecake is a classic dessert loved by almost everyone. But oh—the cream cheese, eggs, and buttery graham cracker crust! Here, we swap a few ingredients for a delicious cheesecake that is airy and creamy, without excess calories and fat.

1 (10-ounce) jar sugar-free jam (such as Polaner All Fruit with Fiber or Smucker's)

1¼ cups Fiber One cereal

24 ounces fat-free cream cheese

2 (16-ounce) cartons Egg Beaters 100% Egg Whites

10 packets nonnutritive sweetener

- Preheat the oven to 350 °F.
- Combine the sugar-free jam with the cereal, and spread the mixture in a nonstick quiche dish (approximately 11 inches in diameter).
- In a blender, mix the cream cheese, egg whites, and nonnutritive sweetener. Pour the mixture on top of the cereal.
- Bake for 40 minutes.

SERVES 18

The Miracle Carb Diet Nutritional Content for Journaling

Per serving: 6 g carbohydrate, 3 g fiber

Actual Nutritional Content

Per serving: 98 calories, 16 g carbohydrate, 3 g fiber, 10 g protein, 1 g fat, 0 g sat. fat, 224 mg sodium

APPLE CRUMBLE

Whenever I visit my grandma's home, I'm greeted by the intoxicating aroma of Apple Crumble baking in the oven. This recipe warms my belly and my heart. Plus, it's a sweet way to get in some extra fiber at the end of dinner.

Nonstick cooking spray

1 cup cracker crumbs (6 high-
   fiber crackers, crushed)

2 teaspoons cinnamon

2 packets nonnutritive
   sweetener

4 Fuji apples, peeled and cored

1 tablespoon lemon juice

- Preheat the oven to 350 °F. Coat a baking dish with nonstick cooking spray. Set aside.
- In a bowl, combine the cracker crumbs, cinnamon, and nonnutritive sweetener. Chop the apples and place them evenly across the baking dish. Sprinkle with the lemon juice.
- Spread the crumble mixture evenly on top of the apples.
- Bake for 30–40 minutes, or until apples are soft.

   SERVES 4

The Miracle Carb Diet Nutritional Content for Journaling
Per serving: 24 g carbohydrate, 10 g fiber

Actual Nutritional Content
Per serving: 72 calories, 25 g carbohydrate, 10 g fiber, 3 g protein, 0 g total fat, 0 g sat. fat, 1.5 mg sodium

BREAKFASTS

CREAMY MOCHA SMOOTHIE

As soon as warm weather hits, I'm overcome with a craving for this frosty coffee blend. However, most coffee shop varieties contain more calories than an entire meal. With my recipe, you can get your cold and creamy mocha fix without the extra calories.

1 (6-ounce) container fat-free plain Greek yogurt

1 cup coffee, already made

½ cup cracker crumbs (3 high-fiber crackers, crushed)

2 teaspoons unsweetened cocoa powder

½ teaspoon cinnamon

Add all the ingredients to a blender and blend until smooth.

SERVES 2

The Miracle Carb Diet Nutritional Content for Journaling
Per serving: 12 g carbohydrate, 8 g fiber

Actual Nutritional Content
Per serving: 74 calories, 15 g carbohydrate, 8 g fiber, 12 g protein, 0 g total fat, 0 g sat. fat, 35 mg sodium

BANANA SMOOTHIE

Smoothies can be a delicious way to get in essential vitamins and minerals, but be sure to choose your smoothies wisely! An original Banana Berry smoothie from Jamba Juice sounds innocent enough, but packs in a whopping 400 calories, 1.5 grams of fat, and 94 grams of carbohydrate. This smoothie recipe is just what you need for a nutrition boost in the morning.

1 (6-ounce) container fat-free plain Greek yogurt

½ cup cracker crumbs (3 high-fiber crackers, crushed)

1 small banana

2 tablespoons Nestlé Coffee-Mate Vanilla Caramel Sugar Free Liquid

½–1 cup ice, according to preference of thickness

Add all ingredients to a blender and blend until smooth.

SERVES 1

The Miracle Carb Diet Nutritional Content for Journaling
Per serving: 38 g carbohydrate, 17 g fiber

Actual Nutritional Content
Per serving: 224 g calories, 48 g carbohydrate, 20 g fiber, 25 g protein, 1 g fat, 0 sat. fat, 84 mg sodium

LEO SCRAMBLE

What does LEO stand for? Well, lox, eggs, and onions, of course! This is a scrumptious twist on your standard scrambled eggs. It's simple to prepare, delicious to eat, and packed with protein. Forget the fork—scoop up this scramble with a high-fiber cracker!

Nonstick cooking spray

1 small onion, thinly sliced

½ teaspoon salt

½ teaspoon pepper

8 ounces lox, chopped

1 dozen egg whites

3 tablespoons skim milk

16 high-fiber crackers

- Spray a large skillet with nonstick cooking spray. Heat over medium-high heat. Add the onion, salt, and pepper, and sauté about 2–3 minutes, until the onions are soft. Add the lox, and sauté for 1 minute.
- In a bowl, beat the egg whites and skim milk with a fork until frothy. Slowly pour the egg whites into the pan. When the eggs have set on the bottom, scramble until just set. Serve with high-fiber crackers.

   SERVES 4

The Miracle Carb Diet Nutritional Content for Journaling
Per serving: 2 g carbohydrate, 1 g fiber

Actual Nutritional Content
Per serving: 135 calories, 12 g carbohydrate, 1 g fiber, 23 g protein, 2 g total fat, 0 g sat. fat, 974 mg sodium

SWEET RICOTTA WITH CRACKERS AND BERRIES

Who says you can't have dessert for breakfast? Creamy chocolate ricotta and fresh berries make the perfect filling for two high-fiber crackers. The perfect mix of fiber and protein in one sweet breakfast sandwich!

½ cup fat-free ricotta

2 packets nonnutritive sweetener

½ teaspoon vanilla extract

1 teaspoon unsweetened cocoa
   powder

¼ cup berries (raspberries, blueberries)

4 high-fiber crackers

Mix the fat-free ricotta, nonnutritive sweetener, vanilla extract, and cocoa powder together in a bowl. Evenly distribute the ricotta mixture on two high-fiber crackers, add berries, and then top each with a high-fiber cracker to form a sandwich.

   SERVES 2

The Miracle Carb Diet Nutritional Content for Journaling
Per serving: 17 g carbohydrate, 11 g fiber

Actual Nutritional Content
Per serving: 131 calories, 26 g carbohydrate, 11 g fiber, 13 g protein, 0 g total
    fat, 0 g sat. fat, 117 mg sodium

MEXICAN OMELET WITH SALSA

*Huevos rancheros, or "ranch-style eggs," is a classic Mexican dish. Layered
with black beans, fresh salsa, and low-fat cheese, this is a delicious meal to
sink your teeth into.*

Nonstick cooking spray

1 medium onion, chopped

½ cup red bell pepper, diced

1 large tomato, chopped

½ cup canned black beans,
    rinsed and drained

1 teaspoon salt

8 egg whites

¼ cup reduced-fat shredded
    Cheddar cheese

½ teaspoon pepper

½ cup chunky salsa, to serve

2 high-fiber crackers
    (optional)

- Spray a medium pan with nonstick cooking spray, and place on medium-
  high heat. Add the onion and pepper, and sauté for about 2 minutes,
  until soft. Add the tomato and beans, and cook until heated through.
  Then remove the mixture from the pan and set aside in a bowl.
- Spray the pan again with nonstick cooking spray, add the egg whites,
  and cook over medium-high heat until the egg whites begin to set.
- Add the shredded Cheddar and pour the vegetable mixture to one side
  of the egg whites. Once the egg whites are set enough, use a spatula to
  flip over the plain half of the egg whites to create an omelet. Serve with
  2 high-fiber crackers, if desired.
- Serve with a side of salsa.

    SERVES 2

The Miracle Carb Diet Nutritional Content for Journaling
Per serving: 10 g carbohydrate, 7 g fiber

Actual Nutritional Content
Per serving: 210 calories, 26 g carbohydrate, 7 g fiber, 23 g protein, 3 g total
fat, 1 g sat. fat, 694 mg sodium

SALADS AND STARTERS

EDAMAME SALAD

Edamame isn't just for when you're having sushi. It makes a great side dish, too; edamame is the only vegetable that offers a complete protein profile equal to both meat and eggs. Edamame is rich in calcium, iron, zinc, and many of the B vitamins.

6 cups water

1 teaspoon salt

3 cups (about 1 bag) frozen shelled edamame (such as Seapoint Farms)

3 cups fresh spinach leaves

1 cup cucumber, chopped

1 cup red bell pepper, seeded and chopped

1 cup radish, sliced

2 tablespoons rice vinegar

1 teaspoon sesame oil

1 tablespoon low-sodium soy sauce

1 teaspoon ginger root, peeled and finely grated

¼ teaspoon pepper

- Combine the water and ½ teaspoon salt in a large saucepan. Bring to a boil.
- Add the edamame. Reduce heat to medium, and boil gently, uncovered, for 5 minutes.
- Rinse with cold water and drain well. Transfer the edamame to a large bowl.
- Add the spinach leaves, cucumber, pepper, and radish to the bowl.

- Whisk the remaining ingredients in a small bowl, and add to the spinach and edamame mixture. Toss to coat and serve.

SERVES 6

The Miracle Carb Diet Nutritional Content for Journaling
Per serving: 0 g carbohydrate, 4 g fiber

Actual Nutritional Content
Per serving: 104 calories, 8 g carbohydrate, 4 g fiber, 5 g protein, 5 g total fat, 0 g sat. fat, 501 mg sodium

LENTIL SALAD WITH SALMON

Lentil salad is a perfect, light, and refreshing dish any day of the week and especially so in the hot summer months. I love adding salmon to bump up the omega-3s and to make this into a healthy, filling meal.

Nonstick cooking spray
4 (4-ounce) fresh salmon
   fillets
2 teaspoons salt
½ tablespoon pepper
1 large red bell pepper, seeded
   and chopped
1 large green bell pepper, seeded
   and chopped

1 large cucumber, skinned and
   chopped
1 red onion, finely chopped
2 cups low-sodium canned
   lentils
2 teaspoons Dijon mustard
2 tablespoons olive oil
3 tablespoons lemon juice

- Preheat the oven to 425 °F. Spray a baking sheet with nonstick cooking spray.
- Season the salmon with salt and pepper. Place the salmon on the prepared baking sheet, and bake for approximately 25 minutes.
- After the salmon is cooked, flake the salmon with a fork. Chill the salmon in the refrigerator while you prepare the lentil salad.

- Add the chopped peppers, cucumber, onion, and lentils to a large bowl and mix.
- In a small bowl, mix the mustard, olive oil, and lemon juice. Add the salmon to the vegetables, and drizzle the salad with the dressing. Mix together gently until the ingredients are evenly incorporated.

SERVES 6 (1 CUP PER SERVING)

The Miracle Carb Diet Nutritional Content for Journaling
Per serving: 13 g carbohydrate, 7 g fiber

Actual Nutritional Content
Per serving: 260 calories, 21 g carbohydrate, 7 g fiber, 22 g protein, 9 g fat, 1 g sat. fat, 133 mg sodium

COBB SALAD

Just because something is called a "salad" doesn't make it good for you. For example, a California Pizza Kitchen Cobb Salad packs in more than 1,000 calories and 85 grams of fat! My recipe for the classic Cobb swaps out full-fat ingredients for a salad both your taste buds and waistline can enjoy.

3 tablespoons white wine vinegar

2 tablespoons shallot, finely minced

1 tablespoon Dijon mustard

¼ teaspoon salt

1 teaspoon pepper

¼ cup nonfat Greek yogurt

1 tablespoon water

4 slices turkey bacon

8 cups (about 2 heads) romaine lettuce, thinly sliced

2 cups (about 1 pound) poached or grilled chicken breast, diced

2 cups cherry tomatoes, halved

2 hard-boiled eggs, peeled and quartered, yolks removed

1 large cucumber, seeded and sliced

1 firm, ripe avocado, pitted, peeled, and thinly sliced

2 ounces low-fat bleu cheese, crumbled

- Whisk together the vinegar, shallot, mustard, salt, and pepper. Blend with the yogurt and the water, and whisk until smooth. Set aside.
- Cook the turkey bacon according to package directions, stirring frequently until crisp. Remove from heat and let cool, then chop into ¾-inch pieces. Set aside.
- Arrange the lettuce on a large platter. Scatter the bacon on top of lettuce, followed by the chicken, tomatoes, egg whites, cucumber, avocado, and low-fat bleu cheese. Drizzle with the dressing or serve on the side.

Tip: To poach the chicken, place the boneless, skinless chicken breasts in a medium skillet or saucepan and add lightly salted water to cover and bring to a boil. Cover, reduce heat to low, and simmer gently until chicken is cooked through and no longer pink in the middle, 10–15 minutes.

SERVES 8

The Miracle Carb Diet Nutritional Content for Journaling
Per serving: 0 g carbohydrate, 7 g fiber

Actual Nutritional Content
Per serving: 263 calories, 14 g carbohydrate, 7 g fiber, 17 g protein, 14 g total fat, 3 g sat. fat, 288 mg sodium

HOMEMADE GARLIC AND HERB HUMMUS

Make this hummus for a delicious afternoon snack! You can reap the benefits of chickpeas by making your own hummus and skipping the large quantities of oil and tahini most brands use. Homemade hummus is super simple and quick to make!

1 (15-ounce) can low-sodium chickpeas

1 tablespoon olive oil

½ cup fresh parsley, stems removed and chopped

2 tablespoons lemon juice

3 cloves garlic, chopped   1 teaspoon cumin

1 teaspoon ground chili pepper

Combine all the ingredients in a food processor or blender. Blend until smooth. Serve and enjoy!

SERVES 4

The Miracle Carb Diet Nutritional Content for Journaling

Per serving: 20.5 g carbohydrate, 6 g fiber

Actual Nutritional Content

Per serving: 217 calories, 23 g carbohydrate, 6 g fiber, 7 g protein, 12 g total fat, 2 g sat. fat, 188 mg sodium

BABA GHANOUSH

This Mediterranean dip is another favorite whenever guests arrive. Serve with toasted whole wheat pita or crudités for a delicious crunch. Eggplant sops up oil like a sponge, so I've removed the oil from this recipe. This dish is best when refrigerated 3 hours before serving.

2 eggplants   1 teaspoon onion powder

2 tablespoons lemon juice   ¼ teaspoon cumin

5 cloves garlic, minced and   ½ teaspoon parsley, chopped
  preferably roasted (see tip
  below)

- Preheat the oven to 400 °F.
- Slice the eggplants in half and pierce with a fork in several places. Set on a baking pan and roast for about 45 minutes, or until soft. Allow to cool slightly, and then scoop out the inside of the eggplants, discarding the skin.
- In a blender or food processor, process the eggplant with the remaining ingredients until smooth.

Tip: To roast garlic, place garlic cloves unpeeled onto a sheet of aluminum foil and gather the sides to create a little pouch. Roast in the oven at 400 °F for 20 minutes, or until the garlic is soft. Once the garlic is cool enough to handle, simply squeeze the garlic out from the skin.

SERVES 4

The Miracle Carb Diet Nutritional Content for Journaling
Per serving: 13 g carbohydrate, 8 g fiber

Actual Nutritional Content
Per serving: 65 calories, 16 g carbohydrate, 8 g fiber, 3 g protein, .5 g total fat, 1 g sat. fat, 6 mg sodium

SOUPS

WHITE BEAN AND ESCAROLE SOUP

This is one of my favorite soups because it is so warm and filling and is always great for family dinners. White Bean and Escarole Soup is a perfect example of a traditional Italian main course. Escarole is a common green used in Italian cooking and is loaded with nutrients such as fiber and folate.

2 tablespoons olive oil

3 cloves garlic, chopped

4 cups low-sodium chicken or vegetable broth

1 pound escarole, chopped

1 large red bell pepper, seeded and chopped

1 (15-ounce) can cannellini beans

½ tablespoon pepper

2 teaspoons salt

- Pour the olive oil in a large pot on medium heat. Add the garlic and sauté about 2 minutes, until slightly browned.
- Add the chicken or vegetable broth, escarole, and red pepper. Simmer

for about 5 minutes, then add the cannellini beans. Allow to simmer for an additional 20 minutes, or until soup is heated through.

- Season with salt and pepper, and serve.

SERVES 4

The Miracle Carb Diet Nutritional Content for Journaling
Per serving: 15 g carbohydrate, 5 g fiber

Actual Nutritional Content
Per serving: 225 calories, 25 g carbohydrate, 5 g fiber, 10 g protein, 11 g total fat, 2 g sat. fat, 815 mg sodium

SPLIT PEA SOUP

Who doesn't like Split Pea Soup? Well, if you think you don't, please try this recipe!

2 cups (about 1 pound) split peas, rinsed	1 onion, finely chopped
6 cups cold water	3 cloves garlic, finely chopped
5 cups chicken broth	1 teaspoon dried thyme
1 carrot, peeled and finely chopped	2 bay leaves
1 stalk celery with leaves, finely chopped	1 tablespoon salt
	2 teaspoons pepper

- In a Dutch oven or soup pot, bring the peas and water to a boil. Reduce heat, cover, and simmer for 2 hours, stirring occasionally.
- Add the remaining ingredients to the pot. Cover and simmer for 30 minutes, or until peas are soft and soup has thickened.
- Remove the bay leaves. Cool slightly and serve.

SERVES 8

The Miracle Carb Diet Nutritional Content for Journaling
Per serving: 10 g carbohydrate, 4 g fiber

Actual Nutritional Content
Per serving: 70 calories, 12 g carbohydrate, 4 g fiber, 5 g protein, 1 g total fat, 0 g sat. fat, 570 mg sodium

LENTIL SOUP

Lentils are packed with fiber and protein, which is why I eat this soup three, four, maybe five times a week. I love it because it never leaves you feeling hungry but at the same time won't weigh you down. Enjoy a warm bowl of this nutritionally packed soup anytime.

Nonstick cooking spray

2 onions, chopped

1 carrot, peeled and diced

1 celery stalk, chopped

2 cloves garlic, minced

1 teaspoon fresh ginger, peeled and grated

½ tablespoon salt

6 cups beef or chicken stock

2 cups red lentils

1 (14.5-ounce) can diced tomatoes

1½ teaspoons ground coriander

½ teaspoon ground cardamom

½ teaspoon ground cumin

- Spray nonstick cooking spray into a large 6-quart pot, and heat over medium heat. Once hot, add the onions, carrot, celery, garlic, ginger, and salt. Sauté until the onions are translucent, approximately 6–7 minutes.
- Add the remaining ingredients, and stir to combine.
- Simmer for 30 minutes or until lentils are soft.

SERVES 8

The Miracle Carb Diet Nutritional Content for Journaling
Per serving: 15 g carbohydrate, 5 g fiber

Actual Nutritional Content

Per serving: 170 calories, 20 g carbohydrate, 5 g fiber, 9 g protein, 5 g total fat, 1 g sat. fat, 380 mg sodium

ITALIAN MINESTRONE SOUP

Minestrone is a great way to start a meal or to eat as a meal on its own! The beans are packed with belly-filling fiber, and the rich tomato broth will keep you coming back for more. This soup fills you up, not out!

Nonstick cooking spray

2 cloves garlic, chopped

1 onion, chopped

2 carrots, chopped

1 cup celery, chopped

2 zucchini, diced

2 cups mushrooms, sliced

1 (14.5-ounce) can cannellini beans

1 (14.5-ounce) can chopped tomatoes

5 cups chicken or vegetable broth

1 teaspoon oregano

1 teaspoon basil

1 tablespoon salt

1 tablespoon black pepper

2 cups frozen spinach, thawed and squeezed dry with a paper towel

½ cup grated Parmesan cheese, to serve

- Spray a large pot with nonstick cooking spray, and heat over high heat. Add the garlic and onion, and sauté until the onion is soft.
- Add the carrots, celery, zucchini, mushrooms, beans, chopped tomatoes, broth, herbs, and seasonings. Bring to a boil. Cover and reduce heat. Simmer for 1 hour. Right before serving, add the spinach and stir.
- Serve topped with grated Parmesan cheese.

    SERVES 6

The Miracle Carb Diet Nutritional Content for Journaling

Per serving: 15 g carbohydrate, 8 g fiber

Actual Nutritional Content

Per serving: 221 calories, 33 g carbohydrate, 8 g fiber, 17 g protein, 5 g total fat, 2 g sat. fat, 766 mg sodium

TURKEY CHILI

Who says chili is just for ski season? By using turkey instead of beef, any chili recipe can be light and filling. You can make a large batch that will last in the freezer for up to 6 months. I like to sprinkle low-fat cheese on top and use high-fiber crackers for dipping.

Nonstick cooking spray

1 pound lean ground turkey breast

1 small onion, chopped, plus more to serve (optional)

3 (15-ounce) cans red kidney beans, drained

3 (14.5-ounce) cans chopped tomatoes

1 cup water

2 celery stalks, chopped

1 medium green bell pepper, seeded and chopped

¼ cup red wine vinegar

2 tablespoons chili powder

2 teaspoons ground cumin

1 teaspoon dried oregano

1 teaspoon dried parsley

1 teaspoon dried basil

Low-fat grated Cheddar cheese, to serve (optional)

Low-fat sour cream, to serve (optional)

- Spray a large pot with nonstick cooking spray, and set over medium heat until hot. Add the ground turkey and onion, and cook until the turkey is browned.
- Add the remaining ingredients, and bring to a boil. Reduce heat to low and simmer uncovered for 30 minutes. Then cover and continue to simmer for another 30–45 minutes, until the chili is thick.

- Serve with low-fat grated Cheddar cheese, onion, or low-fat sour cream, if desired.

SERVES 8

The Miracle Carb Diet Nutritional Content for Journaling
Per serving: 30 g carbohydrate, 13 g fiber

Actual Nutritional Content
Per serving: 282 calories, 39 g carbohydrate, 13 g fiber, 20 g protein, 6 g total fat, 1.5 g sat. fat, 967 mg sodium

POULTRY

CRISPY CHICKEN FINGERS WITH TANGY MUSTARD DIPPING SAUCE

The crispy coating traditionally used for chicken fingers can add a little too much padding around your waistline. Here, with a mixture of seasonings and sliced almonds in place of bread crumbs, you won't miss that fried outer layer one bit. I also remove the majority of the fat content by baking the chicken fingers instead of frying them.

FOR THE CHICKEN FINGERS:

½ teaspoon paprika

2 teaspoons salt

1 teaspoon pepper

⅓ cup sliced almonds

4 (4-ounce) chicken breast fillets

Nonstick cooking spray

FOR THE DIPPING SAUCE:

½ cup orange juice

3 tablespoons Dijon mustard

1½ tablespoons honey

¼ cup water

- Preheat the oven to your broil setting, or around 400–450 °F.
- In a shallow dish, mix together the paprika, salt, pepper, and almonds.

- Coat each chicken breast fillet with almond mixture and place on a Pyrex dish that has been sprayed with nonstick cooking spray.
- Place chicken in oven for about 15 to 20 minutes, turning once halfway through to brown on both sides and cook through.
- While the chicken is cooking, prepare the dipping sauce: In a small bowl, whisk together the orange juice, Dijon mustard, honey, and water until sauce is smooth.

SERVES 4

The Miracle Carb Diet Nutritional Content for Journaling
Per serving: 10 g carbohydrate, 1.0 g fiber

Actual Nutritional Content
Per serving: 311 calories, 14 g carbohydrate, 1 g fiber, 37 g protein, 12 g total fat, 2 g sat. fat, 427 mg sodium

CHICKEN SATAY

When my son Tobey went away to sleepaway camp, the one thing he requested on visiting day was chicken satay from Philippe restaurant. Now that he's back home, I often make my little satay lover my own version of this dish. It also makes a great appetizer at parties!

1 teaspoon garlic, finely chopped

1 teaspoon salt

¼ teaspoon white pepper

2 tablespoons reduced-sodium soy sauce

1 tablespoon dark molasses

2 teaspoons fresh lime juice

2 pounds boneless, skinless chicken breasts cut into strips

Nonstick cooking spray

- Combine the garlic, salt, and pepper in a deep bowl, and mash them to a paste with the back of a spoon.
- Mix in the soy sauce, molasses, and lime juice. Add the chicken strips

and toss until they are evenly coated. Marinate in the refrigerator for 2 hours, stirring occasionally.

- Preheat the broiler.
- Remove the chicken from the marinade and thread it on small skewers (preferably Oriental wooden skewers about 6 inches long).
- Spray chicken evenly with nonstick cooking spray. Cook under the kitchen broiler for 5–10 minutes, turning occasionally, until the chicken is crisp and brown.

SERVES 8

The Miracle Carb Diet Nutritional Content for Journaling
Per serving: 2g carbohydrate, 0g fiber

Actual Nutritional Content
Per serving: 166 calories, 2g carbohydrate, 0g fiber, 26g protein, 4g total fat, 0g sat. fat, 424mg sodium

TURKEY PICCATA

This turkey dish is downright irresistible. Forget about frying—this lemony turkey is golden and delicious without all the extra butter and oil. Enjoy this Italian restaurant favorite at home with a glass of white wine and a fresh garden salad.

Nonstick cooking spray

1 pound turkey, cut into 4 cutlets

1 clove garlic, crushed

1 tablespoon (about ½ lemon) lemon juice

½ cup dry white wine

1 tablespoon capers, chopped

1 teaspoon salt

3 tablespoons fresh or dried parsley, chopped

- Spray a large, heavy skillet with nonstick cooking spray, and set over medium heat. Add the turkey in batches, keeping uncooked pieces from touching. Cook each for 3–4 minutes, until juices run clear.

- Remove the turkey to a platter, and keep warm in the oven or microwave. Using the same skillet, add the garlic, lemon juice, white wine, capers, and salt, and stir around to get the tasty bits off the bottom. Boil for about 1 minute to reduce slightly.
- Put the turkey back into the skillet for another minute, sprinkle the parsley, and serve!

SERVES 6

The Miracle Carb Diet Nutritional Content for Journaling
Per serving: 0 g carbohydrate, 0 g fiber

Actual Nutritional Content:
Per serving: 277 calories, 1 g carbohydrate, 0 g fiber, 32 g protein, 14 g total fat, 3 g sat. fat, 617 mg sodium

TEQUILA LIME CHICKEN

This spicy chicken dish is bright with southwestern flavors. Don't worry about the tequila, either; this festively fun dish only tastes like it's made with what you order at the bar. Actually, it contains no tequila at all.

½ cup fresh lime juice

6 tablespoons soy sauce

2 tablespoons vegetable oil

2 tablespoons fresh oregano, chopped

1 tablespoon fresh rosemary, chopped

1 tablespoon garlic, minced

1½ teaspoons chili powder

½ teaspoon cayenne pepper

8 boneless, skinless chicken breast halves

- Combine all the ingredients (except the chicken) in a medium bowl. Whisk to blend.
- Place the chicken in baking dish. Pour the marinade over the chicken, then cover and refrigerate for 30 minutes, turning occasionally.

- Set the grill to medium-high heat. Remove the chicken breasts from marinade and place on the grill, turning occasionally, until just cooked through, about 10 minutes.
- Transfer the chicken breasts to plates and serve.

SERVES 8

The Miracle Carb Diet Nutritional Content for Journaling
Per serving: 0 g carbohydrate, 0 g fiber

Actual Nutritional Content
Per serving: 190 calories, 6 g carbohydrate, 0 g fiber, 28 g protein, 5 g total fat, 1 g sat. fat, 536 mg sodium

ASIAN LETTUCE CUPS

This dish reminds me of the delicious lettuce wraps at P.F. Chang's but without the extra fat and calories. My whole family loves them and my children love making their own flavorful turkey and lettuce cups.

Nonstick cooking spray

1 large red onion, chopped

1 pound lean ground turkey breast

1 tablespoon soy sauce

1 packet nonnutritive sweetener

¼ cup warm water

½ cup rice vinegar

2 teaspoons chili sauce

2 tablespoons lime juice

1½ cups (about 1 large) cucumber, peeled, seeded, and chopped

⅓ cup fresh mint, coarsely chopped, plus ⅓ cup small mint sprigs

12 large butter lettuce leaves

3 tablespoons hoisin sauce

- Spray a large skillet with nonstick cooking spray, and set over medium-high heat. Add the onion and sauté until beginning to brown, about 3 minutes. Add the turkey and sauté until brown and cooked through, breaking up with the back of a spoon, about 7 minutes.

- In a small bowl, mix together the soy sauce, nonnutritive sweetener, warm water, rice vinegar, chili sauce, and lime juice.
- Add the sauce to the turkey mixture and continue to cook. Stir in the cucumber and chopped mint. Transfer the turkey mixture to a medium bowl. Place the mint sprigs and lettuce leaves on a platter.
- To make the wraps, spread 1 teaspoon of hoisin sauce on each lettuce leaf, then spoon the turkey mixture onto the leaf. Add a few mint sprigs, fold in the sides over the filling, and roll up.

SERVES 4 (3 LETTUCE WRAPS PER SERVING)

The Miracle Carb Diet Nutritional Content for Journaling
Per serving: 0 g carbohydrate, 2 g fiber

Actual Nutritional Content:
Per serving: 234 calories, 15 g carbohydrate, 2 g fiber, 22 g protein, 10 g total fat, 3 g sat. fat, 583 mg sodium

BEEF/PORK/LAMB/VEAL

TEXAS BEEF STEW

The aroma of this hearty Texas Beef Stew alone, simmering on the stove, is enough to whet your appetite. Filled with juicy beef, fresh vegetables, and a rich broth, this delicious stew makes a perfect lunch or dinner for even the hungriest cowboy.

Nonstick cooking spray

3 tablespoons vegetable oil

2 pounds lean beef stew meat, trimmed of fat and cut into 1-inch cubes

2 cups water

2 teaspoons garlic, minced

1 large onion, finely chopped

2 teaspoons chili powder

1 green bell pepper, seeded and chopped

3 cups (about 2 pounds) tomatoes, chopped	1 teaspoon cumin
1 tablespoon oregano	2 cups canned kidney beans

- Coat a large skillet with nonstick cooking spray and place over medium-high heat. Pour in 1½ tablespoons vegetable oil, and brown the meat. Add the water. Simmer covered for 45 minutes, until meat is tender.
- Coat a second skillet with nonstick cooking spray. Add the garlic and onion, and cook over low heat until onion is softened. Add the garlic-onion mixture to the cooked meat. Then add the remaining ingredients to the meat mixture. Simmer for 30 minutes.

Tip: To cut back on sodium, try using "no salt added" canned kidney beans or prepare your own at home without salt.

SERVES 8

The Miracle Carb Diet Nutritional Content for Journaling
Per serving: 13 g carbohydrate, 4 g fiber

Actual Nutritional Content
Per serving: 284 calories, 16 g carbohydrate, 4 g fiber, 33 g protein, 7 g total fat, 0 g sat. fat, 162 mg sodium

BBQ MEATLOAF

Your basic meatloaf just got a little more interesting. The addition of cracker crumbs, onions, and spices, smothered in a tangy barbecue sauce, will make this meatloaf an instant hit. Serve it as a family dinner, and slice up the leftovers for amazing meatloaf sandwiches the next day!

1 pound lean ground beef

½ small onion, finely chopped

½ cup cracker crumbs (3 high-fiber crackers, crushed)

1 egg, lightly beaten

⅔ cup barbecue sauce

Nonstick cooking spray

- Preheat the oven to 350 °F. Combine the ground beef, onion, cracker crumbs, egg, and ⅓ cup barbecue sauce in a large bowl. Shape into a loaf. Wrap in aluminum foil coated with nonstick cooking spray and chill in the refrigerator for 15 minutes.
- Coat a large baking dish with nonstick cooking spray. Place meatloaf mixture in baking dish and shape into loaf.
- Cook meatloaf in oven for 30 minutes, then spoon the remaining ⅓ cup barbecue sauce over the meatloaf. Cook for 15 more minutes to let the sauce caramelize or until meat thermometer inserted into thickest portion reads 155 °F. Serve immediately.

SERVES 6

The Miracle Carb Diet Nutritional Content for Journaling
Per serving: 4 g carbohydrate, 3 g fiber

Actual Nutritional Content
Per serving: 171 calories, 15 g carbohydrate, 3 g fiber, 19 g protein, 5 g fat, 2 g sat. fat, 102 mg sodium

PORK PIZZAIOLA

This easy Italian recipe is a family favorite around my house. Just one bite and you'll understand why. It's like having a delicious pork cutlet topped with your favorite pizza toppings. This recipe is made with tender pork cutlets and fresh vegetables that combine to make a fragrant and flavorful dish.

1 tablespoon olive oil

2 (6-ounce, 1-inch-thick) bone-in pork chops

2 teaspoons salt

½ tablespoon pepper

1 clove garlic, minced

1 small onion, thinly sliced

1 green bell pepper, seeded and cut into strips

1 red bell pepper, seeded and cut into strips

1 cup mushrooms, sliced

¼ teaspoon dried red pepper flakes

1 (15-ounce) can crushed tomatoes

1 tablespoon dried basil

1 tablespoon fresh parsley, chopped finely

- Heat the oil in a heavy, large skillet over medium heat. Season both sides of the pork chops with salt and pepper.
- Add the pork chops to the pan and cook for 4 minutes per side. Transfer the pork chops to a plate and cover with tinfoil to keep them warm. Set aside.
- Next, add the garlic, onion, peppers, and sliced mushrooms to the pan, and sauté over medium-high heat until the vegetables are softened, about 5–7 minutes.
- Add the red pepper flakes, crushed tomatoes, dried basil, and fresh parsley to the skillet.
- Cover the sauce for 15 minutes, until slightly thickened (add a little hot water if sauce becomes too thick). Return the sautéed pork chops to the pan and let cook for 5 minutes, or until pork chops are grilled through.
- Serve each pork chop with pizzaiola sauce and enjoy.

SERVES 2

The Miracle Carb Diet Nutritional Content for Journaling
Per serving: 0 g carbohydrate, 6 g fiber

Actual Nutritional Content
Per serving: 393 calories, 26 g carbohydrate, 6 g fiber, 38 g protein, 15 g fat, 4 g sat. fat, 645 mg sodium

PORK MEDALLIONS WITH MUSHROOM SAUCE

These pork medallions have serious stage presence, making them the center-piece for any dinner party. The mushroom sauce makes it rich and flavorful, just like a delicious Marsala sauce. I serve it with spinach to add a twist on this classic dish.

1 (8-ounce) pork tenderloin
Nonstick cooking spray
1 cup button mushrooms, sliced
   thin
1 clove garlic, minced

1 cup low-sodium beef broth
1 tablespoon fresh rosemary,
   chopped
4 cups fresh spinach leaves

- Slice the tenderloin into ½-inch-thick medallions. Spray a large skillet with nonstick cooking spray, and heat over medium-high heat. Brown the pork for about 2 minutes on each side. Remove from the skillet and set aside.
- Using the same skillet, add the mushrooms and garlic, and sauté for 5 minutes.
- Add the beef broth and fresh rosemary, and bring to a boil, then turn down the heat and simmer until sauce has thickened slightly, about 10 minutes.
- Add the fresh spinach leaves and cover. Cook for 3 minutes, stirring once to wilt the spinach. Place the pork medallions back in the sauce and cook until heated through. Serve.

SERVES 2

The Miracle Carb Diet Nutritional Content for Journaling
Per serving: 0 g carbohydrate, 3 g fiber

Actual Nutritional Content
Per serving: 218 calories, 8 g carbohydrate, 3 g fiber, 30 g protein, 7 g total
   fat, .3 g sat. fat, 171 mg sodium

VEAL PARMIGIANA

I love the veal parmigiana served at my favorite neighborhood Italian restaurant, though I must admit that it comes with more fat and calories than I'd like. My recipe is equally delicious, and it's much lighter because I coat the veal cutlets with cracker crumbs and then bake them in the oven instead of panfrying them.

Nonstick cooking spray

1 large onion, chopped

3 cloves garlic, 2 minced (set aside 1 garlic clove)

1 teaspoon olive oil

½ cup water

4 large tomatoes, chopped

1 teaspoon salt

½ teaspoon pepper

¼ cup fresh basil, chopped

8 veal cutlets

⅓ cup cracker crumbs (2 high-fiber crackers, crushed)

½ teaspoon dried basil

½ teaspoon dried oregano

1 egg white, beaten

2 tablespoons skim milk

1½ tablespoons part-skim mozzarella cheese, shredded

- In a medium saucepan over medium-high heat, sauté the onion and garlic in olive oil until tender. Add the water, tomatoes, salt, and pepper. Bring to a boil and continue to simmer about 10 minutes, or until it reaches desired consistency. Stir in the fresh basil and set aside to keep warm.

- Preheat the oven to 350 °F. Coat a baking dish with nonstick cooking spray.

- Using the flat side of a meat mallet, flatten the veal between two pieces of plastic wrap until they are about ¼ inch thick. Remove from the plastic wrap.

- In a shallow dish, combine the cracker crumbs, dried basil and oregano, and remaining garlic clove. In a small bowl, beat together the egg white and milk. Dip the veal in the egg mixture, then roll in the cracker crumbs.

- Place the coated veal pieces on the prepared baking dish and bake for 20–25 minutes, or until the juices run clear. Transfer the veal to a plate.

- In the same baking dish, layer the bottom with half of the sauce. Place the veal back into the dish, then pour the rest of the sauce over the veal.
- Sprinkle mozzarella cheese over the top, and put back into the oven for another 5–7 minutes, until the cheese melts.

SERVES 8

The Miracle Carb Diet Nutritional Content for Journaling
Per serving: 2 g carbohydrate, 2 g fiber

Actual Nutritional Content
Per serving: 177 calories, 6 g carbohydrate, 2 g fiber, 28 g protein, 5 g total fat, 1 g sat. fat, 657 mg sodium

FISH/SEAFOOD

SEAFOOD SALAD

Frutti di mare, which means "fish of the sea," is a popular dish at many Italian restaurants that comprises a light and refreshing mix of different types of seafood. You don't have to be Italian to make the perfect frutti di mare, though; this recipe is surprisingly simple and always absolutely delicious.

8½ cups water
½ cup Champagne or white wine vinegar
Salt, to taste
1½ pounds (about 25–30) large shrimp, peeled and deveined

1 pound (about 10–12) sea scallops
3 pounds fresh mussels in the shell, scrubbed and debearded

FOR THE SAUCE:
2 tablespoons olive oil

½ teaspoon whole fresh thyme leaves

1 teaspoon fresh garlic, minced

Zest of 2 lemons

¼ cup freshly squeezed lemon
juice

1 teaspoon Dijon mustard

2 tablespoons Champagne or
white wine vinegar

2 teaspoons salt

½ teaspoon pepper

2 stalks celery, diced

1 bunch fresh parsley, chopped

2 lemons, thinly sliced, to
serve

TO MAKE THE SEAFOOD:

• Combine 8 cups water with the Champagne or white wine vinegar and salt in a large saucepan, and bring to a boil.

• Add the shrimp and cook for 2 minutes. Remove with a slotted spoon and set aside.

• Bring the water back to a boil and cook the scallops for 4–5 minutes, until cooked through. Remove the scallops and set aside.

• Drain the saucepan and pour in ½ cup of water. Bring to a boil and toss in the mussels. Return to a boil, cover, and steam for 3–5 minutes, until the mussels open. (Discard any that remain unopened after 5 minutes). Drain the saucepan. Carefully remove the mussels from their shells and discard the shells. Drain all the cooked seafood and place in a large bowl.

TO MAKE THE SAUCE:

• Heat the olive oil in a medium sauté pan over low heat, and add the thyme, garlic, and lemon zest. Cook for 1 minute.

• Off the heat, add the lemon juice, mustard, Champagne or vinegar, salt, and pepper.

TO SERVE:

• Pour the hot vinaigrette over the seafood.

• Add the celery and parsley to the bowl, and toss well. This salad can be served immediately, but it is best when allowed to sit, refrigerated, for 1–2 hours. To serve, sprinkle with salt and toss with sliced lemon.

SERVES 6

The Miracle Carb Diet Nutritional Content for Journaling
Per serving: 0 g carbohydrate, 0 g fiber

Actual Nutritional Content
Per serving: 98 calories, 2 g carbohydrate, 0 g fiber, 9 g protein, 5 g total fat,
   1 g sat. fat, 1,381 mg sodium

PAN-SEARED HALIBUT WITH GARLIC AND MUSHROOM BROTH

Halibut is a fish with tons of nutritional value and versatility. This is a fresh and flavorful recipe for any night of the week. The garlic-mushroom broth is rich and fragrant and a totally new twist on always succulent halibut.

Nonstick cooking spray
1 (6-ounce) skin-on halibut fillet
1 cup fish stock
1 cup button mushrooms,
   roughly chopped

6 cloves garlic, minced
½ green mango, julienned
¼ cup enoki mushrooms

- Preheat the oven to 350 °F.
- Spray a large ovenproof sauté pan with nonstick cooking spray, and set over medium-high heat. Place the halibut skin side down in the skillet and sear until slightly crisp, 2–3 minutes.
- Flip the halibut and place the pan into the oven for 6 minutes, or until cooked through.
- Combine the fish stock, button mushrooms, and garlic in a saucepan. Bring to a boil and then reduce to a simmer. Let the broth reduce to about half its volume.
- Add the green mango and enoki mushrooms to the pan, and cook until the enoki mushrooms are soft.

- To serve, place the mushroom sauce on the plate and top with the seared halibut.

SERVES 2

The Miracle Carb Diet Nutritional Content for Journaling
Per serving: 9 g carbohydrate, 3 g fiber

Actual Nutritional Content
Per serving: 125 calories, 16 g carbohydrate, 3 g fiber, 23 g protein, 4 g total fat, 1 g sat. fat, 240 mg sodium

SALMON WITH MAPLE BALSAMIC GLAZE

This scrumptious fish dish can actually help you lose weight! Salmon contains omega-3 fatty acids, which, besides being incredibly healthy, have been shown to boost metabolism. This recipe is quick and simple, and it works just as well with chicken or other seafood.

Nonstick cooking spray
¼ cup sugar-free maple syrup (such as Walden Farms)
1 clove garlic, minced
¼ cup balsamic vinegar

4 (4-ounce) skin-on salmon fillets, patted dry
1 tablespoon salt
¼ teaspoon pepper

- Preheat the oven to 450 °F. Lightly coat a baking pan with nonstick cooking spray.
- In a small saucepan over low heat, mix together the sugar-free maple syrup, garlic, and balsamic vinegar. Heat just until hot and remove from heat.
- Pour half of the mixture into a small bowl to use for basting, and reserve the rest for later.
- Place the salmon skin side down on the baking sheet and season with

salt and pepper. Brush the salmon with the maple syrup mixture. Bake about 10 minutes, brush again with maple syrup mixture, and bake for another 5 minutes. Continue to baste and bake until the fish flakes easily, about 20–25 minutes total.

- Transfer the salmon fillets to plates and top with reserved maple syrup mixture.

    SERVES 4

The Miracle Carb Diet Nutritional Content for Journaling
Per serving: 0 g carbohydrate, 0 g fiber

Actual Nutritional Content
Per serving: 260 calories, 3 g carbohydrate, 0 g fiber, 28 g protein, 14 g total fat, 3 g sat. fat, 67 mg sodium

MARYLAND CRAB CAKES

Who can resist a classic crab cake? Crisp on the outside and filled with tender, sweet crab on the inside, what's not to like—except the fat and calories you get if they happen to be deep-fried. My version calls for broiling rather than frying, which make them refreshingly light with just the right crunchiness.

Nonstick cooking spray
1 cup cracker crumbs (6 high-fiber crackers, crushed)
1 cup low-fat mayonnaise
1 teaspoon prepared brown mustard

2 tablespoons onion, minced
2 tablespoons celery, minced
1 teaspoon Mrs. Dash Original Blend
1 pound (2 cups) crabmeat

- Preheat the broiler. Lightly spray a baking sheet with nonstick cooking spray.
- In a medium bowl, mix together the cracker crumbs, mayonnaise, brown mustard, onion, celery, and Mrs. Dash.

- Gently stir in the crabmeat. Shape into six patties. Place on the prepared baking sheet.
- Broil the crab cakes 8–10 minutes on each side, or until golden brown.

  SERVES 6

The Miracle Carb Diet Nutritional Content for Journaling
Per serving: 7 g carbohydrate, 5 g fiber

Actual Nutritional Content
Per serving: 144 calories, 13 g carbohydrate, 5 g fiber, 11 g protein, 8 g total fat, 1.3 g sat. fat, 205 mg sodium

BLACKENED TILAPIA

Tilapia is so mild and flaky that it works in just about any dish. The only problem is that it can get pretty boring after a while. For a really flavorful twist on tilapia, try giving it a nice blackened char.

1½ tablespoons paprika

1 tablespoon salt

1 tablespoon garlic powder

1 tablespoon onion powder

½ tablespoon pepper

½ tablespoon oregano

1–2 tablespoons olive oil

½ tablespoon cayenne pepper

1 teaspoon thyme

Nonstick cooking spray

4 (4-ounce) tilapia fillets, patted dry

- In a small glass jar or a bowl, combine all the spices. Add the olive oil and whisk to form a paste. Spoon the spice mixture over both sides of the tilapia and rub in with your hands, coating well.
- Coat a large skillet with nonstick cooking spray and heat over medium-high heat. Add the tilapia to the pan, cooking about 3 minutes on each side, or until the fish has become opaque and flakes easily with a fork.

  SERVES 4

The Miracle Carb Diet Nutritional Content for Journaling
Per serving: 0 g carbohydrate, 2 g fiber

Actual Nutritional Content
Per serving: 179 calories, 5 g carbohydrate, 2 g fiber, 24 g protein, 5 g total
     fat, 1 g sat. fat, 1,806 mg sodium

SIDES

BAKED ZUCCHINI FRIES WITH MARINARA SAUCE

I make these zucchini fries for my kids as a healthy alternative to their two favorite snacks: French fries and mozzarella sticks. They are crunchy and even more delicious when dipped in marinara sauce. It doesn't hurt that I love them, too!

Nonstick cooking spray
1 large egg white
1 teaspoon salt
½ teaspoon pepper
⅓ cup cracker crumbs
    (2 high-fiber crackers,
    crushed)

½ teaspoon garlic powder
4 tablespoons grated Parmesan
    cheese
4 medium zucchini, sliced into
    3½-inch sticks
1 cup marinara sauce

- Preheat the oven to 425 °F. Spray a cookie sheet with nonstick cooking spray and set aside.
- In a small bowl, beat the egg white, and season with salt and pepper.
- In a Ziploc bag, place the cracker crumbs, garlic powder, and Parmesan cheese, and shake well to combine.
- Dip the zucchini sticks into the egg, then into the crumb mixture, a few at a time, and shake to coat. Place the coated zucchini in a single

layer on the cookie sheet, and spray more cooking spray on top. Bake for about 20 minutes, or until golden brown.

- Serve with marinara sauce for dipping.

   SERVES 4

The Miracle Carb Diet Nutritional Content for Journaling
Per serving: 3 g carbohydrate, 5 g fiber

Actual Nutritional Content
Per serving: 103 calories, 11 g carbohydrate, 5 g fiber, 10 g protein, 4 g total fat, 3 g sat. fat, 844 mg sodium

JALAPEÑO POPPERS

When it comes to bar food, in my book nothing beats jalapeño poppers. The spiciness of the jalapeño pepper combined with the cool creaminess of the cheese is a taste sensation I just can't resist. While typical poppers are fried, my baked version is just as crispy with the same delicious flavor I can't get enough of.

16 jalapeño peppers
1 cup low-fat cream cheese
6 ounces low-fat Cheddar cheese
4 strips cooked turkey bacon,
   diced
½ teaspoon ground black pepper

1 teaspoon garlic powder
3–4 tablespoons cracker crumbs
   (1½ high-fiber crackers,
   crushed)
2 egg whites, lightly beaten

- Preheat the oven to 475 °F.
- Cut the jalapeño peppers in half lengthwise and remove the seeds. Place cut side up on a baking sheet.
- In a medium bowl, mix the cream cheese, Cheddar cheese, and turkey bacon. Spoon this mixture into the jalapeño pepper halves.

- Mix the black pepper, garlic powder, and cracker crumbs in a zipper-sealed plastic bag.
- Pour mixture onto a shallow plate. One at a time, dip the peppers in the egg white, then roll in the cracker crumbs. Allow 10 minutes to dry.
- Arrange peppers on the baking sheet, and bake until golden brown, about 15 minutes.

SERVES 8

The Miracle Carb Diet Nutritional Content for Journaling
Per serving: 2 g carbohydrate, 3 g fiber

Actual Nutritional Content
Per serving: 194 calories, 13 g carbohydrate, 3 g fiber, 12 g protein, 11 g total fat, 5 g sat. fat, 612 mg sodium

NOT-SO-SOUTHERN GREEN BEANS

Southern foods are known for being robust and filling, and the traditional recipe for southern-style green beans certainly delivers both—plus a pile of calories. This recipe is much lighter because instead of using the standard fatback, bacon, or ham hocks, I spice up my green beans with onions, garlic, black pepper, and crushed red pepper.

1 tablespoon olive oil
1 medium onion, sliced
3 cloves garlic, minced
1 pound green beans (frozen or fresh)

¼ teaspoon salt
¼ teaspoon pepper
¼ teaspoon crushed red pepper flakes

- Heat the olive oil in a large skillet. Add the onion and garlic, and sauté until the onion is tender.
- Add the remaining ingredients, and cover to keep in the steam. Cook

for about 3 minutes. It may be necessary to add a little bit of water (1–2 tablespoons), especially if using fresh green beans.

- Turn the green beans and continue to cook for another 2–3 minutes. Remove the cover of the pan. Finish cooking with the cover off, until the green beans are slightly tender but still crunchy.

SERVES 4

The Miracle Carb Diet Nutritional Content for Journaling
Per serving: 0 g carbohydrate, 1 g fiber

Actual Nutritional Content
Per serving: 70 calories, 8 g carbohydrate, 1 g fiber, 2 g protein, 4 g total fat,
   1 g sat. fat, 293 mg sodium

BALSAMIC ROASTED ASPARAGUS

This is a super-easy side dish that rounds out almost any meal. I like to slightly char the asparagus, which gives it a wonderful crispness. Roasting the asparagus, instead of steaming it, means no more "mushy" spears.

1 pound (about 25 spears)
  asparagus
1 tablespoon olive oil
2 tablespoons balsamic vinegar

½ teaspoon garlic, minced
½ teaspoon salt
½ teaspoon pepper

- Preheat the oven to 425 °F. Line a shallow baking dish or tray with tinfoil.
- Trim off the tough ends of the asparagus spears.
- In a mixing bowl, toss the asparagus with the olive oil, balsamic vinegar, and garlic. Mix until the asparagus is evenly coated.
- Place the asparagus in the baking dish or tray. Sprinkle with salt and pepper.
- Cook until tender, about 12–18 minutes.

SERVES 4

The Miracle Carb Diet Nutritional Content for Journaling
Per serving: 0 g carbohydrate, 2 g fiber

Actual Nutritional Content
Per serving: 53 calories, 4 g carbohydrate, 2 g fiber, 2 g protein, 4 g total fat,
1 g sat. fat, 444 mg sodium

DESSERTS

CINNAMON ROASTED ALMONDS

I love a snack that's sweet and salty at the same time, and this recipe combines both, along with the satisfying crunchiness of roasted almonds.

Nonstick cooking spray

2 egg whites

2 teaspoons pure vanilla extract

4 cups unblanched almonds

2–3 packets nonnutritive
  sweetener

1 teaspoon salt

½ teaspoon ground cinnamon

- Preheat the oven at 300 °F. Coat a baking pan with nonstick cooking spray.
- In a large bowl, beat the egg whites until frothy, then beat in the vanilla. Add the almonds and stir gently to coat.
- Combine the nonnutritive sweetener, salt, and cinnamon. Add to the nut mixture and stir gently to coat.
- Spread the almonds evenly on the prepared baking pan. Bake for 25–30 minutes, or until almonds are crisp, stirring once.
- Cool and store in an airtight container.

SERVES 16

The Miracle Carb Diet Nutritional Content for Journaling
Per serving: 0 g carbohydrate, 4 g fiber

Actual Nutritional Content

Per serving: 208 calories, 7 g carbohydrate, 4 g fiber, 8 g protein, 18 g total
fat, 1 g sat. fat, 159 mg sodium

CREAMY FROZEN STRAWBERRY SORBET

*Traditional sorbet isn't very dieter-friendly. Sure, the fact that it is made
with fruit makes it seem harmless, but what about all that sugar? By using
Greek yogurt and nonnutritive sweetener instead, you get a light, delicious,
refreshing sorbet.*

4 cups whole unsweetened
frozen strawberries

4 tablespoons nonfat Greek
yogurt

2 packets nonnutritive
sweetener

4 sprigs mint, for garnish

- Puree the frozen strawberries in a food processor until crumbly. Let
rest for 30 seconds.
- Add the yogurt and nonnutritive sweetener, and puree until smooth,
scraping down the sides of the food processor.
- Transfer to a 1-quart plastic container, cover, and freeze.
- Before serving, let sit at room temperature for 5 minutes, and garnish
each bowl with a sprig of mint.

SERVES 6

The Miracle Carb Diet Nutritional Content for Journaling
Per serving: 7 g carbohydrate, 2 g fiber

Actual Nutritional Content
Per serving: 36 calories, 8 g carbohydrate, 2 g fiber, 1 g protein, 0 g total fat,
0 g sat. fat, 4 mg sodium

TANGY MANGO SORBET

One spoon of this luscious sorbet will transport you to your very own tropical paradise.

3 cups (about 5–6) ripe mango,
   cubed
1 ripe banana

1 tablespoon orange juice
½ teaspoon lime peel, grated

- Puree the mango and banana in a food processor. Transfer to a small metal bowl. Stir in the orange juice and lime peel, and cover tightly with plastic wrap.
- Freeze until firm, about 2 hours.
- Remove from the freezer, let soften slightly, and beat until smooth in the food processor. Transfer back to the metal bowl and refreeze for 30 minutes.
- Remove from the freezer, let soften slightly, and beat until smooth in the food processor. Serve.

SERVES 12

The Miracle Carb Diet Nutritional Content for Journaling
Per serving: 9 g carbohydrate, 1 g fiber

Actual Nutritional Content
Per serving: 35 calories, 9 g carbohydrate, 1 g fiber, 0 g protein, 0 g total fat, 0 g sat. fat, 1 mg sodium

RASPBERRY TARTLET

One of my best friends created this brilliant recipe that combines my favorite fruit, raspberries, with the creamy smoothness of cheesecake.

Nonstick cooking spray

½ cup cracker crumbs (3 high-fiber crackers, crushed)

1 teaspoon sugar

1–2 tablespoons water

4 ounces low-fat cream cheese

¼ cup nonfat milk

¼ teaspoon vanilla extract

1 cup raspberries

¼ cup Polaner Sugar Free Apricot Preserves with Fiber

SPECIAL EQUIPMENT:

4-cup muffin tin

- Spray four muffin tin cups with nonstick cooking spray.
- In a bowl, mix together the cracker crumbs, cinnamon, and sugar with water (slowly add the water until the mixture becomes the consistency of a graham cracker crust). Press the crumb mixture into each of the muffin tin cups to create a crust.
- In another bowl, add the low-fat cream cheese, milk, sugar, and vanilla extract, and mix thoroughly with a handheld mixer until smooth and creamy.
- Spoon the cream cheese mixture into each muffin tin, and top each tart with ¼ cup raspberries. Refrigerate for 20 minutes so that the tarts are easier to take out of the muffin tin.
- Meanwhile, in a small saucepan, heat the sugar-free apricot spread over medium heat until melted down to a sauce-like consistency. Either spoon or use a cooking brush to glaze the top of each tart with the apricot jam.
- Gently remove each tart by taking a sharp knife and, in a circular motion, going around the tart and carefully popping it out.

    SERVES 4

The Miracle Carb Diet Nutritional Content for Journaling

Per serving: 12 g carbohydrate, 9 g fiber

Actual Nutritional Content

Per serving: 105 calories, 13 g carbohydrate, 9 g fiber, 5 g protein, 5 g total fat, 3 g sat. fat, 148 mg sodium

COCONUT MACAROONS

If you're coco-nuts, then this is the dessert for you. These Coconut Macaroons are the perfect way to satisfy your sweet tooth without going into a sugar coma. They're packed with delicious coconut flavor, yet easy on calories.

3 egg whites at room
   temperature
¼ teaspoon salt
6 packets nonnutritive sweetener

1 teaspoon vanilla extract
1½ cups sweetened coconut
   flakes

- Preheat the oven to 300 °F. Line two cookie sheets with parchment paper and set aside.
- Place the egg whites and salt in the bowl of an electric mixer, and whisk on high speed until they begin to get frothy. Continue whisking, and add half of the nonnutritive sweetener in a steady stream. Add the remaining nonnutritive sweetener, one packet at a time, beating after each addition.
- Remove the egg white mixture from the mixer, and stir in the vanilla and coconut.
- Drop the macaroons in spoonfuls (about half the size of a golf ball) onto the parchment-lined cookie sheet, and bake until they are golden brown, about 20 minutes.

SERVES 12

The Miracle Carb Diet Nutritional Content for Journaling
Per serving: 0 g carbohydrate, 2 g fiber

Actual Nutritional Content
Per serving: 62 calories, 6 g carbohydrate, 2 g fiber, 0 g protein, 4 g total fat, 2 g sat. fat, 106 mg sodium

STAGE THREE

BREAKFASTS

OATMEAL BLUEBERRY PANCAKES

In our house, Sunday mornings mean digging into a stack of fluffy pancakes. To keep things interesting for my kids, I like to change the pancake recipe each week, but this particular one ranks as everyone's hands-down favorite.

2½ cups old-fashioned oats

6 egg whites, beaten

1 cup skim milk

2 teaspoons oil (any kind)

1 teaspoon baking powder

1 teaspoon vanilla extract

1 teaspoon cinnamon

½ cup natural unsweetened
   applesauce

1 cup blueberries

Nonstick cooking spray

- Blend all the ingredients (except the blueberries) in a blender or food processor until fairly smooth (normal pancake mix consistency). Then gently fold the blueberries into the mixture.
- Heat a skillet to medium heat, then coat with nonstick cooking spray.
- Pour ½ cup batter onto the skillet to form each pancake. Cook, flipping once so that each side is a golden-brown color.

SERVES 6

The Miracle Carb Diet Nutritional Content for Journaling
Per serving: 31 g carbohydrate, 4 g fiber

Actual Nutritional Content
Per serving: 194 calories, 31 g carbohydrate, 4 g fiber, 10 g protein, 4 g total fat, 1 g sat. fat, 207 mg sodium

CRUNCHY CINNAMON SWIRL
FRENCH TOAST

Did you ever think you'd see the words crunchy, cinnamon, *and* French toast *used together in a book about losing weight? Well, here they are in a recipe that's as wonderful as it sounds!*

Nonstick cooking spray

⅓ cup egg white

¼ cup skim milk

½ teaspoon vanilla extract

1 cup Kellogg's All-Bran
   Bran Buds cereal, crushed

4 slices of Pepperidge Farm
   100% Whole Wheat
   Cinnamon Swirl Bread with
   Raisins

Sugar-free maple syrup
   (optional)

- Preheat the oven to 400 °F. Spray a baking sheet with nonstick cooking spray.
- Whisk together the egg whites, skim milk, and vanilla extract in a large bowl. Place the crushed cereal in a second bowl.
- Dip both sides of the bread into the egg mixture, and then coat both sides in the crushed cereal (try to coat the bread well).
- Place the bread on the baking sheet. Bake for 8–10 minutes, then flip and bake for another 5–8 minutes, until crispy and cooked thoroughly.
- For a treat, add some sugar-free maple syrup on top if desired.

SERVES 4

The Miracle Carb Diet Nutritional Content for Journaling
Per serving: 29 g carbohydrate, 11 g fiber

Actual Nutritional Content
Per serving: 115 calories, 29 g carbohydrate, 11 g fiber, 5 g protein, 1 g total fat, 0 g sat. fat, 273 mg sodium

SPINACH, ONION, AND CHEESE BREAKFAST WRAP

Nothing gets me going in the morning—and keeps me going until lunch—quite like this egg and cheese breakfast wrap. Easy and convenient, you can enjoy it at home or take it and go!

Nonstick cooking spray

½ Vidalia onion, chopped

1 package fresh spinach

1 dozen egg whites

1 teaspoon salt

½ teaspoon pepper

4 wedges Laughing Cow Light Garlic & Herb cheese, crumbled

4 whole wheat tortillas

- Heat a nonstick skillet over medium-low heat, and spray with nonstick cooking spray.
- Add the onion and sauté until translucent, approximately 3 minutes.
- Add the spinach and cook until the spinach is wilted.
- Season the egg whites with salt and pepper, and beat vigorously with fork.
- Pour the egg whites over the vegetables, and mix thoroughly.
- Sprinkle Laughing Cow cheese over the top when egg whites are almost set, and mix well with ingredients to scramble.
- Cook until eggs are done and put in tortillas. Roll up and serve immediately.

SERVES 4

The Miracle Carb Diet Nutritional Content for Journaling
Per serving: 10 g carbohydrate, 10 g fiber

Actual Nutritional Content
Per serving: 177 calories, 19 g carbohydrate, 10 g fiber, 21 g protein, 4 g total fat, 1 g sat. fat, 900 mg sodium

CINNAMON BLUEBERRY MUFFIN

Dessert for breakfast? Yes, please! Satisfy your Saturday-morning sweet tooth guilt-free with a healthy and delicious Cinnamon Blueberry Muffin.

Nonstick cooking spray

1¼ cups whole wheat flour

¼ teaspoon salt

1 tablespoon baking powder

½ teaspoon cinnamon

½ teaspoon nutmeg

1½ cups Kellogg's All-Bran Bran Buds cereal

1¼ cups skim milk

2 egg whites

½ cup honey

¼ cup canola oil

1 teaspoon lemon peel, grated

1 cup blueberries

SPECIAL EQUIPMENT:

12-cup muffin tin

- Preheat the oven to 400 °F. Lightly spray a muffin tin with nonstick cooking spray.
- Stir together the flour, salt, baking powder, cinnamon, and nutmeg.
- In a large bowl, mix the cereal and milk. Let the mixture stand for 2 minutes to allow the cereal to soften.
- Beat the egg whites, and add to the cereal mixture. Add the honey, canola oil, and lemon peel, and stir to combine. Add the blueberries, then the dry ingredients, and stir until mixed.
- Pour the batter into the muffin tin and bake for 20 minutes.

SERVES 12

The Miracle Carb Diet Nutritional Content for Journaling

Per serving: 29 g carbohydrate, 5 g fiber

Actual Nutritional Content

Per serving: 157 calories, 29 g carbohydrate, 5 g fiber, 4 g protein, 5 g total fat, 0 g sat. fat, 195 mg sodium

BANANA BERRY SMOOTHIE

Bananas and berries, oh my! This tasty, refreshing breakfast drink has enough protein and fiber to keep you feeling full until lunch.

⅓ cup raspberries

⅓ cup blueberries

⅓ cup blackberries

½ ripe banana

1 5.3 oz. container fat-free Greek yogurt

1 cup ice

In a blender, combine all the ingredients. Blend until smooth and frothy. Pour into a glass and enjoy.

SERVES 2

The Miracle Carb Diet Nutritional Content for Journaling

Per serving: 13 g carbohydrate, 4 g fiber

Actual Nutritional Content

Per serving: 69 calories, 14 g carbohydrate, 4 g fiber, 4 g protein, 0 g total fat, 0 g sat. fat, 10 mg sodium

SALADS AND STARTERS

SESAME NOODLES

This recipe should come with a warning sign, because it is downright addictive. I've cut the calories and fat in this noodle dish by more than half by ditching traditional peanut butter and using PB2 instead. Enjoy these noodles cold for lunch or warm as a side dish.

1 (7-ounce) box whole wheat
 noodles

2 tablespoons PB2

1 packet nonnutritive
 sweetener

Pinch cinnamon

1 tablespoon water

½ tablespoon low-sodium
 soy sauce

2 teaspoons sesame seeds

1 teaspoon garlic, minced

2 teaspoons salt

1 teaspoon pepper

2 tablespoons scallions, chopped

- Cook the noodles according to the instructions on the package.
- Meanwhile, in a separate small dish, prepare the PB2 by mixing it with the nonnutritive sweetener, cinnamon, and water. Once combined, add the soy sauce, sesame seeds, garlic, salt, and pepper. Mix well.
- Drain the noodles once cooked. Pour the sauce over the noodles, mixing thoroughly.
- Top with chopped scallions, and mix again. Chill in the fridge or serve warm.

SERVES 6

The Miracle Carb Diet Nutritional Content for Journaling
Per serving: 23 g carbohydrate, 4 g fiber

Actual Nutritional Content
Per serving: 122 calories, 24 g carbohydrate, 4 g fiber, 1 g protein, 1 g total fat, 0 g sat. fat, 263 mg sodium

VEGETABLE RISOTTO

It's hard to say no to a bowl of creamy, decadent risotto. The problem is that risotto is basically a big bowl of rice, meaning lots of carbs. Plus, add in the butter and cheese and you are looking at a heart attack on a plate. Not to worry: By using barley and loading up on veggies, I have created a risotto-like dish that would fool even the best chef!

8 cups low-sodium chicken broth

1 tablespoon olive oil

1 small onion, finely chopped

10 ounces white mushrooms, finely chopped

2 cloves garlic, minced

1 cup pearl barley

⅔ cup dry white wine

¾ cup frozen peas, thawed

2 cups cooked asparagus, trimmed and cut into 1-inch pieces

½ cup grated Parmesan cheese

½ teaspoon salt

2 teaspoons pepper

- In a heavy medium saucepan over low heat, bring the broth to a simmer. Keep the broth over very low heat.
- In a heavy saucepan over medium heat, add the olive oil. Add the onion and cook until tender, about 5 minutes.
- Add the white mushrooms and garlic, and sauté until the mushrooms are tender and juices evaporate, about 5 minutes.
- Stir in the barley, and let it toast for a few minutes.
- Add the wine, and cook until liquid is absorbed, stirring often, about 2 minutes.
- Add one cup of hot broth to the saucepan. Simmer over medium-low heat until the liquid is absorbed, stirring often, about 3 minutes.
- Continue to cook until the barley is just tender and the mixture is creamy, adding more broth by cupfuls and stirring often, about 20 minutes.
- Stir in the peas and asparagus, and mix in the Parmesan cheese.
- Season with salt and pepper, and serve.

SERVES 8

The Miracle Carb Diet Nutritional Content for Journaling
Per serving: 22 g carbohydrate, 6 g fiber

Actual Nutritional Content
Per serving: 219 calories, 29 g carbohydrate, 6 g fiber, 12 g protein, 5 g total fat, 2 g sat. fat, 416 mg sodium

MEDITERRANEAN COUSCOUS

I love Mediterranean food, and couscous always comes to mind when I am craving this fare. This recipe can be served hot for a satisfying dinner side or cold for a refreshing, zesty summer salad. Try this delicious couscous for a quick fix that pairs well with any meal.

1 cup water

¾ cup instant whole wheat
    couscous

½ teaspoon salt

⅛ teaspoon pepper

4 ounces low-fat feta cheese

2 tablespoons fresh lemon juice

2 cups zucchini, diced

2 cups red bell pepper, diced

1 cup cucumber, diced

1 cup fresh corn kernels

1 tablespoon fresh parsley, finely
    chopped

1 teaspoon green onions,
    chopped

- Bring the water to a boil in a 1-quart heavy saucepan. Stir in the couscous, salt, and pepper, then cover the pan and remove from heat. Let stand, covered, for 5 minutes.
- Fluff the couscous with a fork, and stir in the remaining ingredients.
- Enjoy this salad warm or cold.

    SERVES 8

The Miracle Carb Diet Nutritional Content for Journaling
Per serving: 18 g carbohydrate, 3 g fiber

Actual Nutritional Content
Per serving: 125 calories, 23 g carbohydrate, 3 g fiber, 5 g protein, 2 g total fat, 1 g sat. fat, 105 mg sodium

WHEAT BERRY SALAD

A wheat berry is not a berry at all but a delicious whole grain with a crunch. They are loaded with nutrients and just as easy to prepare as rice. This warm wheat berry salad makes a perfect lunch or side dish. After all, isn't it time you tried something new?

1 cup uncooked wheat berries

2 medium green apples, chopped

1 orange, peeled and thinly sliced

1 stalk celery, chopped

1 red bell pepper, seeded and chopped

¼ cup walnuts, chopped

½ cup Craisins or dried cranberries

½ red onion, chopped

¼ cup apple cider vinegar

2 tablespoons red wine vinegar

3 tablespoons fresh orange juice

2 tablespoons fresh lemon juice

½ teaspoon salt

2 teaspoons pepper

¼ cup fresh mint leaves, chopped, or 2 tablespoons dried mint leaves (optional)

- Place wheat berries in a medium-size pot and cover with at least 2 inches of water. Set aside on your counter, uncovered, to let soak 6–8 hours or overnight. Drain well.
- Transfer pot to stove and bring to a boil. Cover and reduce heat to medium-low. Let wheat berries simmer for one hour or until tender. (Wheat berries retain a firm, chewy texture when cooked.) Drain and set aside to cool.
- Transfer the wheat berries to a large bowl. Add all the ingredients to the bowl. Mix together and serve at room temperature, or you can refrigerate it for up to 1 week.

SERVES 8

The Miracle Carb Diet Nutritional Content for Journaling
Per serving: 22 g carbohydrate, 3 g fiber

Actual Nutritional Content

Per serving: 125 calories, 25 g carbohydrate, 3 g fiber, 3 g protein, 3 g total fat, 0 g sat. fat, 156 mg sodium

GRILLED TEX-MEX SALAD

When my husband, Glenn, orders a taco salad, I am not fooled into thinking he is making a healthy choice. I know he is really aching for that crispy, crunchy tortilla that accompanies the salad as a bowl. This Grilled Tex-Mex Salad is a great way to spice up your traditional tossed salad. All the usual taco fillings are turned inside out with corn as the base. Spices such as chili powder and cumin turn up the heat a bit and may help with weight loss and improve your immune system.

FOR THE SALAD:

4 ears corn, husked with the silk removed

½ cup onion, finely chopped

1 can black beans, rinsed and drained

1 jalapeño pepper, chopped (retain the seeds if you like it hot)

1 red bell pepper, seeded and chopped

1 cup cherry tomatoes, halved

FOR THE DRESSING:

½ cup lime juice

2 teaspoons olive oil

1 teaspoon mild chili powder

½ teaspoon cumin

½ teaspoon salt

¼ teaspoon pepper

- Place the corn on the grill and roast, turning often, until golden brown on the outside. (You may also boil the corn instead.)
- When the corn cools, cut the kernels off into a bowl.
- Add the onion, beans, jalapeño, pepper, and tomatoes, and set aside.
- Combine all the dressing ingredients in a small bowl. Pour over the

corn mixture and toss. Let sit in the refrigerator for an hour, or overnight, before serving.

SERVES 4

The Miracle Carb Diet Nutritional Content for Journaling
Per serving: 20 g carbohydrate, 9 g fiber

Actual Nutritional Content
Per serving: 279 calories, 36 g carbohydrate, 9 g fiber, 10 g protein, 11 g total
fat, 0 g sat. fat, 703 mg sodium

SOUPS

BEEF AND BARLEY SOUP

*This soup always reminds me of being at my grandma Claire's house. She
would always have a big pot of this soup waiting for me when I arrived. It
is rich and hearty and full of flavor. Thanks, Grandma Claire, for always
loving me!*

Nonstick cooking spray

2 (8-ounce) packages sliced
   mushrooms (feel free to mix
   up your mushroom selection)

1 medium onion, chopped

1 medium carrot, peeled and
   finely chopped

½ cup celery, finely chopped

1 tablespoon garlic, minced

12 ounces lean beef stew meat,
   cut into bite-size pieces

6 cups reduced-sodium beef or
   vegetable broth

2 cups water

2 teaspoons salt

1 teaspoon pepper

2 sprigs fresh thyme

1 cup uncooked barley

2 tablespoons fresh parsley,
   chopped

- Heat a pan over medium-high heat. Coat the pan with nonstick cooking spray. Add the mushrooms and onion, and sauté for 10 minutes, or until lightly browned. Spoon the onion mixture into a medium bowl.
- Recoat the pan with cooking spray. Add the carrot, celery, and garlic, and sauté for 4 minutes, or until lightly browned. Combine the carrot mixture with the onion and mushrooms in the bowl.
- Spray a large pot with nonstick cooking spray, and place over medium-high heat. Add the beef and cook for 3 minutes, browning on all sides.
- Add 1 cup broth to the pan, scraping the bottom of the pot to loosen browned bits. Add the remaining broth, onion and carrot mixture, water, salt, pepper, and thyme.
- Bring to a boil, then cover and reduce heat to medium-low. Simmer for 1 hour, or until beef is just tender.
- Discard the thyme sprigs. Stir in the barley, cover, and cook for 30 minutes, or until the barley is al dente. Uncover and cook an additional 15 minutes. Remove from heat. Sprinkle with parsley and serve.

SERVES 8

The Miracle Carb Diet Nutritional Content for Journaling
Per serving: 17 g carbohydrate, 5 g fiber

Actual Nutritional Content
Per serving: 206 calories, 24 g carbohydrate, 5 g fiber, 16 g protein, 6 g total fat, .2 g sat. fat, 130 mg sodium

CHICKEN AND CORN CHOWDER

From a dietitian's point of view, chowder translates into lots of cream and lots of fat headed straight to your waistline. Swapping the cream with a spicy tomato base saves on fat and calories while adding a zesty surprise kick! In combination with a hint of sweetness from the corn, this soup translates into a delicious and healthy choice for any day of the week.

4 ears corn

2 cups water

4 cups reduced-sodium chicken broth

1 carrot, peeled and chopped

1 onion, chopped

1 tablespoon salt

1 teaspoon thyme

1 teaspoon peppercorns

2 boneless, skinless chicken breasts, cut into chunks

Nonstick cooking spray

1 can Tex-Mex–style tomatoes

1 teaspoon cumin

1 teaspoon paprika

1 teaspoon garlic powder

1 teaspoon cilantro

- Slice off the corn kernels and set aside in a bowl. Place the ears into a large pot with the water and chicken broth.
- Add the carrot, onion, salt, thyme, and peppercorns. Bring to a boil and allow to simmer for 30 minutes.
- Carefully strain the stock to remove the corn ears and discard. Return the stock to your pot.
- Add the diced chicken, and bring back up to a simmer.
- In a skillet sprayed with nonstick cooking spray, add the corn kernels and sauté until just starting to brown. Add the corn to the stockpot.
- Add the remaining ingredients to the stockpot. Simmer for half an hour, or until chicken is cooked through.

SERVES 8

The Miracle Carb Diet Nutritional Content for Journaling
Per serving: 15 g carbohydrate, 3 g fiber

Actual Nutritional Content
Per serving: 161 calories, 21 g carbohydrate, 3 g fiber, 17 g protein, 3 g total fat, 1 g sat. fat, 909 mg sodium

BUTTERNUT SQUASH SOUP

Butternut Squash Soup reminds me of everything I love about the fall. The delicious spice and sweetness of this recipe will warm you up when the weather starts to get cold. No need to add cream—pureeing this soup gives it a silky, creamy consistency no one will be able to resist!

3 cups (about 1 pound) butternut squash, peeled, seeded, and cubed

Nonstick cooking spray

1 tablespoon fresh ginger, peeled and grated

1 large onion, chopped

3–4 cloves garlic, chopped

1 cup carrots, peeled and diced

4 cups chicken stock

2–3 teaspoons ground ginger

⅔ teaspoon salt

⅛ teaspoon pepper

2–3 teaspoons cinnamon

- Preheat the oven to 350 °F.
- Spray the cubes of butternut squash with nonstick cooking spray, and spread onto a baking sheet. Bake for 40 minutes, or until soft, and remove from the oven.
- Place a large soup pot over medium-low heat, and add the fresh ginger, onion, and garlic, and cook for a couple of minutes.
- Add the squash, carrots, chicken stock, ground ginger, salt, and pepper. Bring to a boil, then reduce heat and simmer with the lid on for 20–30 minutes, or until the carrots are tender.
- Carefully pour the soup into a blender, and blend the soup until it is thick and there are no large chunks. Transfer the soup back to the heated soup pot, and stir in the cinnamon.

SERVES 6

The Miracle Carb Diet Nutritional Content for Journaling
Per serving: 8 g carbohydrate, 3 g fiber

Actual Nutritional Content

Per serving: 84 calories, 17 g carbohydrate, 3 g fiber, 5 g protein, 1 g total fat, 0 g sat. fat, 970 mg sodium

VEGETABLE SOUP

Sautéed vegetables add a delicious layer of flavor to this soup and boost the vitamin and mineral content. Sautéing the vegetables allows them to cara-melize, giving them a robust flavor.

Nonstick cooking spray

²⁄₃ cup carrot, peeled and sliced

½ cup onion, diced

2 cloves garlic, minced

3 cups low-sodium beef, chicken, or vegetable broth

⅓ cup celery, chopped

1½ cups green cabbage, diced

½ cup green beans

1 (10-ounce) can diced tomatoes with green chilies (mild or hot)

2 teaspoons salt

1 teaspoon pepper

½ cup zucchini, diced

½ teaspoon dried basil

¼ teaspoon dried oregano

- Spray a large saucepan with nonstick cooking spray, and place over low heat.
- Sauté the carrot, onion, and garlic until softened, about 5 minutes.
- Add the broth, celery, cabbage, green beans, tomatoes, salt, and pepper, and simmer, covered, for about 15 minutes, or until beans are tender.
- Stir in the zucchini and cook for 3–4 minutes. Add the basil and oregano. Serve.

SERVES 6

The Miracle Carb Diet Nutritional Content for Journaling

Per serving: 0 g carbohydrate, 4 g fiber

Actual Nutritional Content

Per serving: 60 calories, 11 g carbohydrate, 4 g fiber, 4 g protein, 1 g total fat, 0 g sat. fat, 142 mg sodium

CHICKEN NOODLE SOUP

This is a take on my grandma Claire's chicken vegetable soup. It's chock-full of chunks of white meat chicken and hearty vegetables, and the whole wheat noodles add extra fiber and comfort. Warm up in the cold winter months with a bowlful of this soup. One bite and you will be hooked.

Fresh parsley, 1 bunch

Fresh dill, 1 bunch

6 chicken breasts

2 cups water

4 cups chicken broth

4 carrots, peeled and halved

2 turnips, peeled and halved

2 parsnips, peeled and halved

2 stalks celery, halved

1 leek, halved

½ teaspoon salt

2 teaspoons pepper

1 cup whole wheat egg noodles

SPECIAL EQUIPMENT:

Cheesecloth

- Wrap the parsley and dill in the cheesecloth.
- Place the chicken breasts in a large pot over medium-high heat. Cover with the water and chicken broth.
- Add the cheesecloth containing the parsley and dill, along with the rest of the ingredients. Bring to a boil, then lower heat and simmer for 1 hour, adding the whole wheat egg noodles when there are 20 minutes left.
- Remove and discard the cheesecloth containing the herbs.
- Carefully remove and shred the chicken and dice the vegetables, then return them to the soup. Heat to a simmer and serve.

Tip: You can skim the soup by putting it in the refrigerator and letting the fat layer congeal, then removing it.

SERVES 8

The Miracle Carb Diet Nutritional Content for Journaling
Per serving: 11 g carbohydrate, 2 g fiber

Actual Nutritional Content
Per serving: 138 calories, 22 g carbohydrate, 2 g fiber, 19 g protein, 0 g total fat, 0 g sat. fat, 200 mg sodium

POULTRY

SWEET AND SOUR MEATBALLS

I love re-creating retro dishes, such as the popular party appetizer Sweet and Sour Meatballs. My kids always request these meatballs for dinner, which are sweet just like them!

1 (12-ounce) can or bottle chili sauce
2 teaspoons lemon juice
1 (10-ounce) jar Polaner All Fruit with Fiber Grape Spreadable Fruit
1 pound lean ground turkey breast
1 egg, beaten
1 large onion, grated
½ cup cracker crumbs (3 high-fiber crackers, crushed)
¼ teaspoon salt

- Whisk together the chili sauce, lemon juice, and grape jelly. Pour into a saucepot and simmer over low heat.
- Combine the remaining ingredients in a large bowl. Mix well and form into 1-inch balls. Add to the sauce and simmer for 45 minutes.

SERVES 4

The Miracle Carb Diet Nutritional Content for Journaling
Per serving: 5 g carbohydrate, 10 g fiber

Actual Nutritional Content
Per serving: 400 calories, 52 g carbohydrate, 10 g fiber, 26 g protein, 10 g total fat, 11 g sat. fat, 126 mg sodium

CHICKEN AND RED ONION QUESADILLAS

This is a flavor-packed quesadilla that will blow you away. It's got the crunch, cheese, and kick—who can ask for more? Olé!

2 small red onions, thinly sliced
½ cup balsamic vinegar
Nonstick cooking spray
6 whole wheat tortillas

1½ cups shredded low-fat
    Cheddar cheese
1 pound boneless chicken
    breast, cooked and shredded

- Combine the onions and vinegar in a bowl, and allow to marinate for 5 minutes. Drain the onions and set aside.
- Spray a large skillet with nonstick cooking spray, and heat over medium heat. Add the marinated onions, and cook until onions have softened, about 5–7 minutes. Transfer onions to a bowl and set aside until ready to stuff the quesadillas.
- Place 2 tortillas in a large nonstick skillet over medium-high heat (they will overlap). Warm for about 45 seconds, then flip to warm the other side.
- Sprinkle ¼ cup of cheese on each tortilla. Cover cheese with the shredded cooked chicken, and top the chicken with one-sixth of the marinated onions.
- Fold the tortillas in half, press gently with a spatula to flatten, and cook for about 2 minutes, until the cheese begins to melt. Flip the quesadilla and cook for another 1–2 minutes, until the second side is golden.
- Transfer to a plate and cover with foil to keep warm. Serve warm.

SERVES 3 (2 QUESADILLAS PER SERVING)

The Miracle Carb Diet Nutritional Content for Journaling
Per serving: 20 g carbohydrate, 15 g fiber

Actual Nutritional Content
Per serving: 413 calories, 36 g carbohydrate, 15 g fiber, 53 g protein, 11 g
total fat, 4 g sat. fat, 715 mg sodium

TURKEY AND BLACK BEAN NACHOS

Find the free tortilla chips at Mexican restaurants hard to resist? Keep in mind that every 15 chips equals 200 calories. That's why I make my own fiesta at home with this delicious and healthy Turkey and Black Bean Nachos recipe.

Nonstick cooking spray
2 tablespoons olive oil
1 pound ground turkey breast
1 cup onion, chopped
1 clove garlic, pressed
¾ teaspoon cumin

¼ teaspoon salt, plus more to
taste
2 (15-ounce) cans black beans
10 corn tortillas
Pepper, to taste
1 jar pico de gallo, to serve

- Preheat the oven to 400 °F. Spray a baking sheet with nonstick cooking spray and set aside.
- Heat the oil in a skillet. Add the ground turkey and chopped onion. Sauté until the meat is cooked through. Add the garlic and seasonings, blend, and simmer for 10 minutes or more to allow flavors to blend. Add the beans to the turkey mixture, and cook on low heat for 5 minutes. Set aside.
- Spray each tortilla with nonstick cooking spray, and sprinkle with salt and pepper. Using a knife or pizza cutter, cut each tortilla into eight triangles to create chips.
- Place the chips onto the prepared baking sheet. Bake the chips for 15 minutes, or until golden brown and crispy.

- Serve topped with ground turkey mixture and pico de gallo.

  SERVES 8

The Miracle Carb Diet Nutritional Content for Journaling
Per serving: 11 g carbohydrate, 4 g fiber

Actual Nutritional Content
Per serving: 210 calories, 12 g carbohydrate, 4 g fiber, 14 g protein, 12 g total
   fat, 2 g sat. fat, 125 mg sodium

CHIMICHURRI CHICKEN

Can't think of anything new to do with chicken? This Latin-inspired recipe
offers a twist that will have your family begging for more!

FOR THE SAUCE:

3 tablespoons olive oil

1/3 cup red wine vinegar

1/2 cup low-sodium chicken or
   vegetable broth

4 cloves garlic

1 shallot, sliced

1 tablespoon lemon juice

1/4 cup cilantro

2 tablespoons parsley, chopped

1 teaspoon oregano

1 teaspoon basil

1/2 teaspoon coarse salt

1/2 teaspoon pepper

FOR THE CHICKEN:

4 (4-ounce) boneless, skinless
   chicken breasts

Nonstick cooking spray

TO MAKE THE SAUCE:

- Place all the ingredients in a food processor and blend until combined.
- Let flavors marry by setting aside for at least 20–30 minutes at room
  temperature.
- Remove 45 minutes before serving to bring the sauce to room temperature.

TO MAKE THE CHICKEN:

· Preheat the oven to 350 °F.

· Place the chicken in a baking dish sprayed with nonstick cooking spray. Lightly spray the chicken with nonstick cooking spray.

· Bake for 25–30 minutes, or until center is no longer pink or juices run clear.

· Plate the chicken and pour ¼ cup chimichurri sauce onto each breast.

SERVES 4

The Miracle Carb Diet Nutritional Content for Journaling
Per serving: 0 g carbohydrate, 1 g fiber

Actual Nutritional Content
Per serving: 225 calories, 8 g carbohydrate, 1 g fiber, 22 g protein, 6 g total fat, 2 g sat. fat, 330 mg sodium

PESTO CHICKEN

Pesto no longer needs to be tossed with a bowlful of spaghetti. It is a great addition that adds a ton of flavor to any dish.

12 ounces cooked chicken breasts
4 tablespoons Fresh Basil Pesto
  (see page 159)
Nonstick cooking spray
1 cup arugula leaves
1 cup mesclun mix
1 clove garlic, crushed

¼ cup sun-dried tomatoes, chopped
1½ cups broccoli florets, steamed until tender
½ cup almonds, blanched and slivered
½ red onion, thinly sliced

· Preheat the oven to 400 °F.

· Slather the cooked chicken breasts with pesto sauce, place on a baking sheet coated with nonstick cooking spray, and bake for about 5 minutes, until bubbly and slightly browned.

- Remove from the oven, chop chicken into bite-size pieces, and place in a large mixing bowl.
- Add the remaining ingredients to the bowl. Toss and serve.

SERVES 6 (APPROXIMATELY ⅔ CUP PER SERVING)

The Miracle Carb Diet Nutritional Content for Journaling
Per serving: 0 g carbohydrate, 7 g fiber

Actual Nutritional Content
Per serving: 175 calories, 7 g carbohydrate, 7 g fiber, 17 g protein, 9 g total fat, 1 g sat. fat, 311 mg sodium

BEEF/PORK/LAMB/VEAL

BEEF BRISKET

Brisket is always the star at any of my holiday get-togethers, and my mother's recipe is always a showstopper. Her secret? Ketchup that gives the brisket a sweetness that makes it a guaranteed crowd-pleaser.

1 tablespoon vegetable oil	2 cloves garlic, peeled and
1 (3-pound) beef brisket	halved
Black pepper	1 cup ketchup
4 onions, thickly sliced	

- Heat the oil in a large, deep skillet or pot over medium-high heat. Season the brisket generously with black pepper. Place in the pan and cook until the bottom and sides are a rich brown color, not burned, but dark. Lift the roast and scatter the onions in the pan. Place the uncooked side of the roast down onto the onions. Repeat the browning process.
- Add the garlic and ketchup to the pan, and fill with enough water to almost cover the roast. Bring to a simmer. Reduce heat to low and cover with a lid or tight-fitting aluminum foil. Simmer for 4 hours,

turning the roast over once halfway through. The roast should be fork tender.

- Remove the brisket to a serving platter. Bring the broth in the pan to a simmer, scraping the bottom to loosen any browned bits. Cook until reduced to a thin gravy, and serve alongside the brisket.

SERVES 12

The Miracle Carb Diet Nutritional Content for Journaling
Per serving: 0 g carbohydrate, 1 g fiber

Actual Nutritional Content
Per serving: 385 calories, 10 g carbohydrate, 1 g fiber, 21 g protein, 29 g total fat, 1 g sat. fat, 294 mg sodium

LAMB AND EGGPLANT STEW

The lamb in this dish was inspired by my favorite Turkish restaurant in the city. I have frequented this restaurant so many times I was able to re-create this recipe with all the taste but with fewer calories. It is full of flavor and light enough to be eaten all year round.

Nonstick cooking spray

4 medium cloves garlic, finely chopped

1 medium onion, chopped

2 pounds extra lean lamb, trimmed of all fat and cut into large chunks (this should leave about 1¼ pounds)

2 cups beef stock

1 eggplant, peeled and cut into cubes

1 (6-ounce) can tomato paste

3 tablespoons apple juice

2½ tablespoons lemon juice

1 teaspoon cinnamon

1 tablespoon fresh ginger, peeled and chopped

1 teaspoon ground coriander

½ teaspoon salt

½ teaspoon pepper

2 tablespoons fresh cilantro, chopped

- In a 4-quart saucepan sprayed with nonstick cooking spray, sauté the garlic and onion over medium heat for 2–3 minutes.
- Add the lamb chunks and ¼ cup beef stock, and cook for 5 minutes over medium heat, stirring occasionally.
- Add the eggplant and remaining stock, and cook for 5 minutes over medium-low heat.
- Stir in the tomato paste, apple juice concentrate, lemon juice, cinnamon, ginger, ground coriander, salt, and pepper. Cover and cook on low heat for 25 minutes. Add the fresh cilantro, and cook for 5 more minutes.

SERVES 6

The Miracle Carb Diet Nutritional Content For Journaling
Per serving: 0 g carbohydrate, 6 g fiber

Actual Nutritional Content
Per serving: 325 calories, 26 g carbohydrate, 6 g fiber, 27 g protein, 8 g total fat, 2 g sat. fat, 430 mg sodium

LAMB SOUVLAKI

Lamb Souvlaki is a soft and tender Greek dish. I serve these juicy chunks of lamb in a whole wheat pita with fresh vegetables. The cool, creamy F-Factor Tzatziki Sauce adds a rich creaminess to these perfect pitas.

Juice of ½ lemon

1 tablespoon olive oil

1 tablespoon fresh garlic, chopped

1½ teaspoons oregano

¼ teaspoon pepper

¼ teaspoon salt

1 pound lamb, cut into 16 equal-size cubes

1 red onion, cut into 8 pieces

2 yellow bell peppers, cut into bite-size pieces

2 green bell peppers, cut into bite-size pieces

16 cherry tomatoes

Nonstick cooking spray

4 whole wheat pitas, to serve

F-Factor Tzatziki Sauce, to serve

- In a large bowl, mix together the lemon juice, olive oil, garlic, oregano, black pepper, and salt. Add the lamb, onion, bell peppers, and tomatoes, and stir to coat. Cover and refrigerate for 30 minutes.
- Heat a nonstick grill pan sprayed with nonstick cooking spray over medium-high heat. Thread the lamb, peppers, onion, and tomatoes onto skewers, using four pieces of lamb per skewer.
- Cook for 10–15 minutes, or to desired doneness, turning the skewers frequently for even cooking.
- Serve with the whole wheat pitas and F-Factor Tzatziki Sauce.

  SERVES 4

The Miracle Carb Diet Nutritional Content for Journaling

Per serving: 15 g carbohydrate, 6 g fiber

Actual Nutritional Content

Per serving: 390 calories, 32 g carbohydrate, 6 g fiber, 25 g protein, 19 g total fat, 7 g sat. fat, 416 mg sodium

F-FACTOR TZATZIKI SAUCE

When you think of Mediterranean foods, dishes such as hummus and baba ghanoush may immediately come to mind. Have you ever tried Tzatziki? This light and flavorful sauce is truly delicious and it complements a wide variety of dishes. Note: Tzatziki sauce can be kept covered in the refrigerator for up to one week. It actually tastes better the second day!

1 (16-ounce) container plain
  nonfat Greek yogurt
2 lemons, juiced (about ½ cup)
½ cup flat leaf parsley, minced
¼ cup fresh dill, minced

2 large cucumbers, peeled and
  minced
1 teaspoon salt
1 teaspoon pepper

Prepare Tzatziki sauce by mixing in a large bowl, Greek yogurt, lemon juice, parsley, dill, cucumbers, and salt and pepper. Refrigerate for 15–30 minutes.

SERVES 4

The Miracle Carb Diet Nutritional Content for Journaling
Per Serving: 15 g carbohydrate, 6 g fiber

Actual Nutritional Content
Per Serving: 390 calories, 32 g carbohydrate, 6 g fiber, 25 g protein, 19 g total fat, 7 g sat. fat, 516 mg sodium

F-FACTOR CHEESEBURGER

You don't have to go to the drive-thru to enjoy a burger. Try my recipe to truly get burgers done your way. You'll save yourself money, time, and a lot of extra calories!

¾ pound 90% lean ground beef
¾ pound lean ground turkey
  breast
¼ cup barbecue sauce
2 teaspoons salt
1 teaspoon pepper
6 slices low-fat Cheddar cheese

6 lettuce leaves
6 (½-inch-thick) slices tomato
6 multigrain buns, split and
  toasted
Ketchup (optional)
Low-fat mayonnaise (optional)
Sliced pickles (optional)

- Prepare a charcoal or gas grill.
- Mix together the beef, turkey, and barbecue sauce, and form into six 4-ounce patties. Add salt and pepper.
- Grill for approximately 7–8 minutes on each side for medium to medium-well burgers. Just before the burgers are done, top with a slice of cheese.
- Place the lettuce and tomato on the top half of a bun, and place the burger on top. Cover with the other half of the bun. Serve with condiments such as ketchup, mayonnaise, or pickles, if desired.

SERVES 6

The Miracle Carb Diet Nutritional Content for Journaling
Per serving: 36 g carbohydrate, 4 g fiber

Actual Nutritional Content
Per serving: 345 calories, 42 g carbohydrate, 4 g fiber, 37 g protein, 8 g total fat, 2 g sat. fat, 602 mg sodium

STEAK FAJITAS

Steak Fajitas can be a healthy and satisfying dinner. Instead of filling your tortilla with fattening condiments, add bulk to your meal with peppers and onions. Now you can enjoy Mexican food without looking like an overstuffed piñata.

1 pound flank steak, trimmed of any fat
1 clove garlic, minced
½ teaspoon chili powder
½ teaspoon dried oregano, crushed
4 whole wheat tortillas
Nonstick cooking spray

1 medium onion, sliced
1 medium green bell pepper, seeded and cut into thin strips
1 large tomato, chopped
¼ cup salsa
½ cup lettuce, shredded
¼ cup nonfat sour cream

- Preheat the oven to 350 °F.
- Slice the beef into thin strips. Toss with garlic, chili powder, and oregano.
- Wrap the tortillas in foil and place in the oven.
- Spray a pan with nonstick cooking spray. Add the onion and pepper, and cook for 1½ minutes. Remove the vegetables from the skillet.
- Add the beef strips and cook until desired doneness. Drain off any fat. Add the tomato and cooked onion and peppers.
- Fill the warm tortillas with beef mixture and top with salsa, lettuce, and sour cream. Serve immediately.

SERVES 4

The Miracle Carb Diet Nutritional Content for Journaling
Per serving: 10 g carbohydrate, 10 g fiber

Actual Nutritional Content
Per serving: 255 calories, 28 g carbohydrate, 10 g fiber, 26 g protein, 8 g fat, 2 g sat. fat, 300 mg sodium

FISH/SEAFOOD

FISH TACOS

This is one of my favorite recipes. It reminds me of days spent in Mexico on the beach. The flaky fish works so perfectly with the light and refreshing cucumber slaw. I serve these tacos for lunch, for dinner, at parties . . . basically anywhere I can. They're that good!

FOR THE FISH:

Nonstick cooking spray
½ cup cracker crumbs (3 high-fiber crackers, crushed)
½ teaspoon salt
¼ teaspoon pepper
½ teaspoon garlic powder
2 egg whites, beaten
1 pound cod

FOR THE LIGHT BAJA SAUCE:

¼ cup light mayonnaise

¼ cup fat-free Greek yogurt

¼ teaspoon cayenne pepper

1 tablespoon ketchup

1 tablespoon fresh lime juice

4 La Tortilla Factory Smart & Delicious Low Carb, High Fiber Large Size Tortillas

8 romaine leaves, chopped in strips

- Preheat the oven to 350 °F. Spray a Pyrex dish with nonstick cooking spray.
- In a shallow dish, combine the cracker crumbs, salt, black pepper, and garlic powder. Place the egg whites in a separate dish.
- Cut the cod into four equal pieces. Dip each piece into the egg whites, and then coat evenly with the cracker crumb mix.
- Place the seasoned fish into the Pyrex dish and put in oven for 12–15 minutes, until lightly browned.
- Meanwhile, in a separate bowl, mix all the ingredients for Baja sauce.
- Lay out the tortillas and layer with lettuce strips, one piece of fish, and 2 tablespoons Baja sauce on each.

SERVES 4

The Miracle Carb Diet Nutritional Content for Journaling

Per serving: 15 g carbohydrate, 16 g fiber

Actual Nutritional Content

Per serving: 111 calories, 17 g carbohydrate, 16 g fiber, 12 g protein, 2 g total fat, 0 g sat. fat, 55 mg sodium

SHRIMP SCAMPI WITH WHOLE WHEAT PASTA

Shrimp is one of my favorite proteins to cook with, because it's low in calories and is ready in a snap. Typically shrimp scampi is loaded with butter, but I've skipped the added fat and created this classic with whole wheat pasta and all the other classic ingredients.

1 teaspoon olive oil

¾ pound whole wheat linguine

1½ tablespoons garlic, minced

1 pound (about 16) jumbo shrimp, peeled and deveined

½ teaspoon salt

¼ teaspoon pepper

⅓ cup fresh parsley leaves, chopped

Zest of ½ lemon

¼ cup freshly squeezed lemon juice

⅛ teaspoon hot red pepper flakes

- In a large pot, bring water to boil, then add linguine and cook for 7–10 minutes, or according to the directions on the package.
- Meanwhile, in another large (12-inch), heavy-bottomed pan, heat 1 teaspoon olive oil over medium-low heat. Add the garlic and sauté for 1 minute. (Be careful, the garlic burns easily!)
- Add the shrimp, salt, and pepper, and sauté until the shrimp have just turned pink, about 5 minutes, stirring often.
- Remove from the heat. Add the parsley, lemon zest, lemon juice, and red pepper flakes. Toss to combine.
- Serve the linguine topped with the shrimp.

SERVES 4

The Miracle Carb Diet Nutritional Content for Journaling
Per serving: 37 g carbohydrate, 6 g fiber

Actual Nutritional Content
Per serving: 225 calories, 40 g carbohydrate, 6 g fiber, 14 g protein, 2 g total fat, 0 g sat. fat, 980 mg sodium

CIOPPINO

This fish stew is a favorite of mine whenever I visit the Bay Area. The seafood is combined with tomatoes and wine to make a fragrant broth. Bring a taste of San Francisco into your kitchen with this Cioppino recipe.

1 tablespoon olive oil

1 onion, chopped

1 green bell pepper, seeded and
   chopped

4 cloves garlic, finely chopped

1 cup dry red wine

1 (14-ounce) can diced tomatoes

1 (8-ounce) bottle clam juice

½ cup fresh parsley, chopped

1 bay leaf

½ teaspoon dried oregano

¼ teaspoon crushed red pepper

1 pound mussels

1 pound crab legs, cut into
   4-inch pieces

1 pound medium shrimp, peeled
   and deveined

1 pound firm white fish fillet
   (such as cod, haddock, or
   halibut)

¼ cup fresh basil, chopped

Salt, to taste

Pepper, to taste

- Heat the oil in a heavy pot over medium heat. Add the onion and green pepper, and cook, stirring, until softened, about 5 minutes.
- Add the garlic and cook until aromatic, about 1 minute. Stir in the wine and bring to a boil. Cook for 3 minutes, then add the tomatoes, clam juice, parsley, bay leaf, oregano, and crushed red pepper. Cover, leaving the lid slightly ajar. Simmer, stirring occasionally, until the broth is rich and thick, 20–30 minutes.
- Add the mussels, cover, and cook for 2 minutes. Remove the mussels with tongs as they open, reserving them in a large bowl. Discard any mussels that do not open.
- Add the crab legs and return to a simmer and cook, uncovered, until the crab is heated through, about 5 minutes. Remove with tongs and reserve with the mussels.
- Add the shrimp, fish, and basil. Cover and simmer until the shrimp turns pink and the fish is opaque, 2–3 minutes.

- Discard the bay leaf. Taste and adjust seasonings with salt and pepper. Return the reserved mussels and crab legs to the pot. Reheat briefly and serve.

  SERVES 12

The Miracle Carb Diet Nutritional Content for Journaling
Per serving: 1 g carbohydrate, 2 g fiber

Actual Nutritional Content
Per serving: 260 calories, 12 g carbohydrate, 2 g fiber, 31 g protein, 8 g total fat, 1 g sat. fat, 835 mg sodium

WASABI TUNA BURGER

This is not your basic burger. Seared tuna steak makes up the base, and the spicy hot wasabi sauce adds a kick that's sure to wake up your taste buds.

1 cup low-sodium soy sauce
2 tablespoons green onions, finely chopped

1 teaspoon sugar
4 thin tuna steaks

FOR THE WASABI SAUCE:
4 tablespoons Hellmann's Light Mayonnaise
1 teaspoon water
½ tablespoon wasabi powder or 1 tablespoon prepared wasabi

Nonstick cooking spray
8 tablespoons toasted sesame seeds

- In a small bowl, combine the soy sauce, green onions, and sugar, and mix well.
- Place the tuna in a baking dish and pour the marinade over it. Marinate for at least 15 minutes.

- Meanwhile, in a small bowl, combine all the ingredients for the wasabi sauce and whisk together.
- Spray a cast-iron or heavy-bottomed skillet with nonstick cooking spray, and heat until hot.
- Coat the tuna fillets on all sides with sesame seeds. Cook the tuna for 1–3 minutes on each side, or to desired doneness.
- Serve each tuna burger with a tablespoon of wasabi mayonnaise. Enjoy as either an entrée with a side of vegetables or with a salad.

    SERVES 4

The Miracle Carb Diet Nutritional Content for Journaling
Per serving: 1 g carbohydrate, 4 g fiber

Actual Nutritional Content
Per serving: 422 calories, 13 g carbohydrate, 4 g fiber, 47 g protein, 20 g total fat, 3 g sat. fat, 2,795 mg sodium

SEARED SEA SCALLOPS WITH QUICK AND EASY TOMATO SAUCE

These scallops are seared so that they are crisp on the outside but stay juicy and tender on the inside. I like to serve this dish with a side of sautéed spinach and tomato sauce. Scallops cook quickly, so keep your eye on them when preparing this dish.

Nonstick cooking spray
1½ pounds sea scallops
1 bag fresh spinach

Quick and Easy Tomato Sauce
   (see page 156)

- In a sauté pan, spray and heat nonstick cooking spray. Add the scallops and sear on both sides, about 1–2 minutes per side.
- Remove the scallops from the pan and keep warm until finished making sauce.

- After removing the scallops, add the spinach and cook until wilted, about 5 minutes. Remove from pan and place in a bowl to serve later.
- Add the scallops back to the pan with the Quick and Easy Tomato Sauce and cook another 5 minutes, until scallops are heated and cooked through. Serve with the cooked spinach.

SERVES 6

The Miracle Carb Diet Nutritional Content for Journaling
Per serving: 0 g carbohydrate, 3 g fiber

Actual Nutritional Content
Per serving: 140 calories, 13 g carbohydrate, 3 g fiber, 10 g protein, 3 g total fat, 1 g sat. fat, 1,229 mg sodium

SIDES

SWEET POTATO FRIES

If there is one fried food I can't resist, it's sweet potato fries! They are crunchy, salty, and sweet, my perfect flavor combination. I bake them in the oven for my kids for a crunchy side packed with vitamins and minerals we can all enjoy!

1½ pounds (about 2 large) sweet potatoes

1 teaspoon ground cumin

⅛ teaspoon salt

¼ teaspoon pepper

1 tablespoon olive oil

- Preheat the oven to 400 °F.
- Wash the potatoes and cut each one in half lengthwise. Slice each half into 6–8 long, thin wedges.
- In a large mixing bowl, combine the cut potatoes with the rest of the ingredients, and toss until evenly coated.

- Spread onto a baking sheet and bake for about 40 minutes, or until potatoes are cooked through and edges are slightly crispy.

    SERVES 6

The Miracle Carb Diet Nutritional Content for Journaling
Per serving: 13 g carbohydrate, 5g fiber

Actual Nutritional Content
Per serving: 75 calories, 13 g carbohydrate, 5 g fiber, 1 g protein, 2 g total fat, .5 g sat. fat, 266 mg sodium

HOISIN-GLAZED EGGPLANT

Hoisin sauce is a Chinese sauce that is sweet, salty, and spicy. This sauce used to only be available in specialty markets, but now it's stocked in most major grocery stores. Glazing the eggplant with hoisin makes it sweet and crispy on the outside and soft and creamy on the inside.

¼ cup hoisin sauce

1 teaspoon reduced-sodium soy sauce

2 teaspoons salt, plus more to taste

1 teaspoon pepper, plus more to taste

Nonstick cooking spray

1¼ pounds (about 4 baby or 1 large) eggplant, cut lengthwise into 1-inch-thick slices and scored

- In a small bowl, whisk together the hoisin sauce, soy sauce, salt, and pepper.
- Spray a large skillet or grill pan with nonstick cooking spray, and place on medium-high heat.
- Brush both sides of the eggplant pieces with the hoisin sauce, and season with salt and pepper. Grill until charred and tender, about 5 minutes per side.

- Brush both sides of each eggplant generously with the remaining hoisin mixture, and grill each side again just to glaze, about 1 minute per side. Serve hot.

SERVES 4

The Miracle Carb Diet Nutritional Content for Journaling
Per serving: 13 g carbohydrate, 8 g fiber

Actual Nutritional Content
Per serving: 130 calories, 22 g carbohydrate, 8 g fiber, 2 g protein, 5 g total fat, .5 g sat. fat, 1,888 mg sodium

ZUCCHINI PANCAKE

You don't have to wait for Hanukkah to enjoy latkes during the year. I use zucchini instead of potatoes for a new and nutritious twist on potato pancakes.

1 pound (about 4) medium zucchini	1 teaspoon salt
2 large eggs, lightly beaten	½ teaspoon pepper
6–8 tablespoons all-purpose whole wheat flour	½–1 tablespoon vegetable oil, for frying

- Preheat the oven to 300 °F.
- Grate the zucchini into a large bowl using a grater or a food processor with a grater attachment. Stir in the eggs.
- Stir in 6–8 tablespoons flour until mixture is wet, but not falling apart. Season with the salt and pepper.
- Heat ½ tablespoon oil in a large sauté pan over medium heat. When the oil is hot but not smoking, lower the heat to medium-low and drop heaping soupspoons of batter into the pan. Cook the pancakes about 2 minutes on each side, until browned.

- Place the pancakes on a sheet pan and keep warm in the oven. Wipe out the pan with a dry paper towel, add more oil to the pan, and continue to fry the pancakes until all the batter is used. The pancakes can stay warm in the oven for up to 30 minutes. Serve hot.

SERVES 10

The Miracle Carb Diet Nutritional Content for Journaling
Per serving: 6 g carbohydrate, 3 g fiber

Actual Nutritional Content
Per serving: 69 calories, 10 g carbohydrate, 3 g fiber, 3 g protein, 2 g total fat, .5 g sat. fat, 634 mg sodium

GARLIC MASHED POTATOES

Creamy Garlic Mashed Potatoes are a delicious side to any meal. By leaving the skins on the mashed potatoes and mixing them with skim milk instead of butter, you will add more fiber and cut calories. I love using Greek yogurt instead of sour cream to give it a tangy taste.

2 pounds red bliss potatoes, quartered
8–10 cloves garlic, roasted (see tip on page 228)
⅓ cup plain nonfat Greek yogurt
¼ cup skim milk
1 tablespoon fresh chives
½ teaspoon salt
¼ teaspoon pepper

- Place the potatoes in a large saucepan with enough cold water to cover. Bring to a boil over high heat. Lower heat to maintain a simmer, and cook until tender, about 20 minutes. Drain the potatoes, then return them to the saucepan.
- Mash the potatoes and garlic with a potato masher or an electric mixer on low speed. Add the remaining ingredients. Beat until light and fluffy.

SERVES 6

The Miracle Carb Diet Nutritional Content for Journaling
Per serving: 24 g carbohydrate, 3 g fiber

Actual Nutritional Content
Per serving: 106 calories, 24 g carbohydrate, 3 g fiber, 3 g protein, 0 g total
    fat, 0 g sat. fat, 226 mg sodium

EASY CREAMED SPINACH

I am not a huge steak eater, but when I'm in the mood, I love a yummy creamed spinach side with my juicy steak. Just because it's spinach, though, doesn't mean it's healthy. A standard creamed spinach recipe is weighed down with boatloads of heavy cream. My twist on this classic allows you to get the health benefits of spinach without the heavy cream.

2½ pounds (about 3–4 bunches) flat-leaf spinach, trimmed and cleaned

2 tablespoons butter

½ medium onion, minced

4 cloves garlic, minced

¼ teaspoon salt

1 teaspoon pepper

4 ounces cream cheese

½ cup milk

Pinch ground nutmeg

- Bring a large pot of salted water to a boil. Add the spinach and cook just until wilted, about 1 minute. Drain in a colander and rinse with cold water until cool. Squeeze the spinach to remove as much liquid as possible. Coarsely chop and set aside.
- In a large saucepan, heat the butter over medium heat. Add the onion and garlic, and season with salt and pepper. Cook, stirring occasionally, until the onion softens, 3–5 minutes.
- Add the cream cheese and milk, and cook, stirring, until the cream cheese is melted and smooth. Stir in the spinach. Simmer over me-

dium heat until the mixture thickens, 8–10 minutes. Add the nutmeg and serve.

SERVES 4

The Miracle Carb Diet Nutritional Content for Journaling
Per serving: 2 g carbohydrate, 11 g fiber

Actual Nutritional Content
Per serving: 216 calories, 23 g carbohydrate, 11 g fiber, 17 g protein, 9 g total fat, 5 g sat. fat, 1,395 mg sodium

DESSERTS

CARROT CAKE BITES

Carrot cake is one of my all-time favorite desserts. It's sweet but not too sweet, and I'm a sucker for the cream cheese frosting. By switching out a few ingredients, you can now have your cake and eat it, too.

FOR THE CAKE:

Nonstick cooking spray

½ cup all-purpose flour, plus more for dusting

6 tablespoons whole wheat flour

2 tablespoons oat bran

½ cup Splenda or nonnutritive sweetener

1 teaspoon baking powder

½ teaspoon ground cinnamon

¼ teaspoon baking soda

¼ teaspoon salt

½ cup Egg Beaters

½ cup carrot, finely shredded

4 tablespoons canola oil

¼ cup applesauce

FOR THE FROSTING:

2 ounces reduced-fat cream
cheese

2 ounces Mori-Nu Silken Soft
Tofu

¼ cup fat-free whipped topping

½ cup powdered sugar

½ teaspoon vanilla extract

½ tablespoon orange juice

- Preheat the oven to 350 °F. Grease an 11 × 7 × 2-inch baking dish or a 9-inch square baking dish with nonstick cooking spray. Dust with flour to prevent sticking.
- In a large bowl, stir together the flours, oat bran, nonnutritive sweetener, baking powder, cinnamon, baking soda, and salt. Set aside.
- In another bowl combine the Egg Beaters, carrot, oil, and applesauce. Add this mixture to the flour mixture. Stir until combined. Pour the batter into the prepared pan.
- Bake for 30 minutes, or until a knife inserted into the center comes out clean. Remove from the oven and cool on a wire rack for 10 minutes. Remove from the pan and cool completely.
- Meanwhile, combine all the frosting ingredients in a bowl and mix with an electric mixer until smooth. Frost the cake.
- Cut the cake into 12 pieces and serve.

SERVES 12

The Miracle Carb Diet Nutritional Content for Journaling
Per serving: 16 g carbohydrate, 2 g fiber

Actual Nutritional Content
Per serving: 129 calories, 23 g carbohydrate, 2 g fiber, 3 g protein, 6 g total fat, 1 g sat. fat, 159 mg sodium

CHOCOLATE-COVERED BANANAS

How do you make a banana even better? Cover it in chocolate and stick it in the freezer! Freezing the Chocolate-Covered Banana gives it a Popsicle-like consistency. Hard chocolate coating on the outside and cool creamy banana on the inside!

8 ounces semisweet chocolate, chopped

2 bananas, peeled and cut crosswise into thirds

⅓ cup rainbow sprinkles

SPECIAL EQUIPMENT:
6 Popsicle sticks or wooden skewers

- Place the chocolate in a heatproof bowl set over (not in) a pan of gently simmering water. Stir until melted.
- Line a baking sheet with waxed paper. Insert a Popsicle stick in one end of each banana piece. Dip the banana, one piece at a time, in the chocolate, spooning on additional chocolate to cover.
- Sprinkle each banana with sprinkles, and set on the prepared baking sheet. Freeze until the chocolate is firm, about 20 minutes, or wrap and store up to 3 days.

SERVES 6

The Miracle Carb Diet Nutritional Content for Journaling
Per serving: 36 g carbohydrate, 2 g fiber

Actual Nutritional Content
Per serving: 267 calories, 40 g carbohydrate, 2 g fiber, 2 g protein, 15 g total fat, 9 g sat. fat, 5 mg sodium

CHOCOLATE CHUNK BROWNIES

Sink your teeth into a warm Chocolate Chunk Brownie guilt-free. To cut down on sugar, I've added ingredients that naturally sweeten, such as vanilla and cocoa powder. Once you have your first bite, you'll swear you got 'em from the bake sale down the street!

Nonstick cooking spray

2 (1-ounce) squares unsweetened baking chocolate

¼ cup vegetable oil

¼ cup almond butter

⅔ cup sugar

2 eggs, well beaten

½ teaspoon vanilla extract

¾ cup whole wheat flour

¼ teaspoon salt

½ cup walnuts, chopped

½ cup (about 1) zucchini, grated

- Preheat the oven to 350 °F. Coat an 8-inch square baking dish with nonstick cooking spray.
- In a large saucepan over medium heat, melt the chocolate together with the vegetable oil. Once melted and combined, remove from heat and stir in the remaining ingredients.
- Mix well, and add water, 1 tablespoon at a time, if the batter is too thick to spread.
- Pour the brownie batter into the prepared baking dish. Bake for 25–30 minutes. Remove from the oven, cool, and cut into squares.

SERVES 16

The Miracle Carb Diet Nutritional Content for Journaling
Per serving: 15 g carbohydrate, 2 g fiber

Actual Nutritional Content
Per serving: 152 calories, 15 g carbohydrate, 2 g fiber, 3 g protein, 10 g total fat, 2 g sat. fat, 83 mg sodium

ALMOND COOKIES

Cold weather often entices me to bake. Warming up the kitchen with the heat of the oven and filling my house with the sweet aroma of homemade cookies is the perfect way to wait out the winter weather. However, cookies are high in both sugar and fat, and indulging in a few too many of these treats can add inches to your waistline. With this recipe, you can bake to your heart's content and satisfy even the sweetest tooth.

2 cups almonds, ground   Pinch salt
4 egg whites   1 tablespoon almond extract
½ cup powdered sugar

- Preheat the oven to 350 °F.
- Toast the ground almond on the stove top over low heat, until fragrant. This takes only a few minutes. Set aside to cool.
- In a mixing bowl, combine the egg whites, powdered sugar, salt, and almond extract. Whisk together briskly. Add the cooled almond bits. Combine with the rest of the batter.
- Line a cookie sheet with parchment and spoon the batter onto the paper. The batter will be very runny and rather unruly, so leave plenty of room between the cookies and be gentle when sliding the cookie sheet into the oven.
- Bake for approximately 13 minutes. The cookies should turn a nice golden brown when done. They will also be fragile and a little sticky, so be careful when removing from the parchment.

SERVES 12

The Miracle Carb Diet Nutritional Content for Journaling
Per serving: 7 g carbohydrate, 3 g fiber

Actual Nutritional Content
Per serving: 163 calories, 10 g carbohydrate, 3 g fiber, 6 g protein, 12 g total fat, 1 g sat. fat, 19 mg sodium

CHOCOLATE-CRUNCH-COATED STRAWBERRIES

Delicious, juicy strawberries just got sweeter. I've added a chocolate-covered crunch coating to the outside! I'm using dark chocolate in this recipe instead of milk chocolate for an extra antioxidant boost.

8 ounces semisweet chocolate, chopped

1 pound (about 20) large strawberries, washed and dried well

⅓ cup pistachios, finely chopped

- Place the chocolate in a heatproof bowl set over (not in) a pan of gently simmering water. Stir occasionally until melted, about 3–5 minutes. Remove from heat.
- Line a baking sheet with waxed paper. One at a time, dip each strawberry in chocolate, twirling to coat. Then sprinkle the chocolate-covered portion of the strawberry with pistachios, and place on the waxed paper.
- Chill the chocolate-dipped strawberries at least 15 minutes to set. (Strawberries should not be stored in the refrigerator longer than 1 hour, as condensation drops may collect on the chocolate.)

SERVES 10 (2 STRAWBERRIES PER SERVING)

The Miracle Carb Diet Nutritional Content for Journaling
Per serving: 16 g carbohydrate, 2 g fiber

Actual Nutritional Content
Per serving: 148 calories, 18 g carbohydrate, 2 g fiber, 2 g protein, 8 g total fat, 4 g sat. fat, 2 mg sodium

COCKTAILS

MIXED BERRY DAIQUIRI

Daiquiris are delicious but definitely not low calorie. With tons of added sugar headed straight for your belly, try my recipe to keep your bikini body in shape!

3 ounces Captain Morgan
   Original Spiced Rum
Juice of 1 lime
1 cup frozen strawberries

1 cup raspberries
1 cup ice
2 lime wedges, for garnish

Place the rum, lime juice, strawberries, raspberries, and ice in a blender. Blend until smooth. Pour into two glasses and garnish each rim with a lime wedge.

SERVES 2

The Miracle Carb Diet Nutritional Content for Journaling
Per serving: 16 g carbohydrate, 6 g fiber

Actual Nutritional Content
Per serving: 232 calories, 36 g carbohydrate, 6 g fiber, 2 g protein, 0 g fat, 0 g sat. fat, 2 mg sodium

SUMMER SANGRIA

Summer and fresh fruit go hand in hand. Sangria is a hot weather staple. This recipe is a great way to use red wine collecting dust in your cabinets during the hot summer months.

6 ounces Chalone Pinot Noir

1 ounce brandy

½ cup strawberries, sliced

¼ lime, thinly sliced

¼ lemon, thinly sliced

¼ orange, thinly sliced

¼ apple, peeled, cored, and
sliced

½ cup club soda

½ cup diet ginger ale

- In a chilled pitcher, combine the wine, brandy, and fruit. Refrigerate overnight.
- Remove from the refrigerator, add the club soda and diet ginger ale, pour into glasses filled with ice, and serve.

SERVES 2

The Miracle Carb Diet Nutritional Content for Journaling
Per serving: 14 g carbohydrate, 4 g fiber

Actual Nutritional Content
Per serving: 136 calories, 10 g carbohydrate, 2 g fiber, 0 g protein, 0 g fat, 0 g sat. fat, 34 mg sodium

MUDDLED GINGER AND MINT COOLER

Mint and ginger mix together for a naturally delicious, refreshing drink. Sip poolside or serve at your next summer barbecue to get the neighbors talking!

3 ounces Ketel One Vodka

1 tablespoon ginger, chopped

8 ounces club soda

½ cup mint leaves, muddled

Juice of ½ lime

½ lime, cut into quarters, for
garnish

Combine the vodka, ginger, club soda, mint, and lime juice in a pitcher. Pour into tall glasses with ice, and garnish with lime.

SERVES 2

The Miracle Carb Diet Nutritional Content for Journaling
Per serving: 0 g carbohydrate, 0 g fiber

Actual Nutritional Content
Per serving: 126 calories, 6 g carbohydrate, 0 g fiber, 0 g protein, 0 g fat, 0 g sat.
    fat, 28 mg sodium

MANGO MAI TAI

A classic cocktail with a whole new twist. One sip of this and you'll be looking for the tiki bar and mini umbrellas.

4 ounces Captain Morgan Parrot
    Bay Mango Rum
½ ounce Torani Almond Sugar-
    Free Syrup
½ ounce Teisseire 0% Sugar
    Grenadine Syrup

½ ounce pineapple juice
Juice of 1 lime
Juice of 1 lemon
4 pineapple slices, for garnish
4 mango slices, for garnish

- Scoop ice into a martini shaker until it is half full.
- Pour the rum, syrups, and juices into the shaker, and shake for 30 seconds.
- Pour into glasses filled with ice, and garnish with the pineapple and mango slices.
    SERVES 2

The Miracle Carb Diet Nutritional Content for Journaling
Per serving: 10 g carbohydrate, 2 g fiber

Actual Nutritional Content
Per serving: 186 calories, 16 g carbohydrate, 2 g fiber, 0 g protein, 0 g total
    fat, 0 g sat. fat, 4 mg sodium

BLUEBERRY LEMONADE COCKTAIL

This is my adult play on lemonade. Its flirty, refreshing, and a crowd-pleaser on a hot summer day.

3 ounces Smirnoff Blueberry
   Vodka

1 cup blueberries

2 cups water

1 packet Crystal Light Pure
   Lemonade

1 cup ice

Combine all the ingredients in a blender. Blend until smooth and serve.

SERVES 2

The Miracle Carb Diet Nutritional Content for Journaling
Per serving: 10 g carbohydrate, 2 g fiber

Actual Nutritional Content
Per serving: 132 calories, 10 g carbohydrate, 2 g fiber, 0 g protein, 0 g total
   fat, 0 g sat. fat, 16 mg sodium

KIWI VANILLA COOLER

Who would think to mix kiwi and vanilla? I love Voli Pear Vanilla Vodka and wanted to add a zing with kiwi to set this cocktail apart from the rest.

½ kiwi, peeled

Ice cubes

2 ounces Smirnoff Vanilla
   Vodka

Muddle the kiwi in a mixing glass until well crushed and juicy. Add the ice and vodka, and shake vigorously. Pour all the contents into rock glasses.

SERVES 1

The Miracle Carb Diet Nutritional Content for Journaling
Per serving: 8 g carbohydrate, 0 g fiber

Actual Nutritional Content
Per serving: 143 calories, 8 g carbohydrate, 0 g fiber, 1 g protein, 0 g total fat,
   0 g sat. fat, 1 mg sodium

BASIL BLOODY MARY

*Whenever my associate Rebecca goes to New Orleans, she can't stop raving
about the Bloody Marys. So one day she made her own version for us. Too
good to be kept a secret, here is our NOLA-inspired take on the Bloody Mary.*

3 ounces Moon Mountain
   Organic Vodka
1¼ cups tomato juice
¼ cup fresh basil leaves, finely
   chopped

Juice of 1 lemon
1 teaspoon Worcestershire sauce
1 teaspoon Tabasco Sauce
Pinch black pepper
Celery, for garnish

In a pitcher, combine the vodka, tomato juice, basil, lemon juice, Worcestershire sauce, Tabasco Sauce, and pepper. Pour into glasses filled with
ice, and garnish with a stalk of celery.

SERVES 2

The Miracle Carb Diet Nutritional Content for Journaling
Per serving: 8 g carbohydrate, 0 g fiber

Actual Nutritional Content
Per serving: 140 calories, 10 g carbohydrate, 0 g fiber, 2 g protein, 0 g total
   fat, 0 g sat. fat, 466 mg sodium

RASPBERRY ORANGE SUNRISE

This cocktail is packed full of antioxidants and vitamins and minerals, so drink up—the potassium in the oranges will help keep a hangover at bay.

3 ounces Moon Mountain Wild
    Raspberry Organic Vodka
1 packet Crystal Light Pure
    Tropical Blend

½ cup fresh raspberries
½ cup fresh oranges
Ice

In a blender, combine all the ingredients and blend until smooth. Pour into tall glasses. Sip and enjoy!

SERVES 2

The Miracle Carb Diet Nutritional Content for Journaling
Per serving: 9 g carbohydrate, 3 g fiber

Actual Nutritional Content
Per serving: 142 calories, 9 g carbohydrate, 3 g fiber, 1 g protein, 0 g total fat, 0 g sat. fat, 2 mg sodium

LYCHEE MARTINI

Who doesn't love Mr. Chow's famous lychee martini? My skinny jeans! I still love Mr. Chow's, but I must drink responsibly—for my waistline.

3 ounces Ketel One Vodka
2 ounces Naked Juice Reduced
    Calorie Lychee

Splash vermouth
Ice
4 fresh lychees

Combine the vodka, lychee juice, and vermouth. Pour over ice. Garnish with two lychees per glass.

SERVES 2

The Miracle Carb Diet Nutritional Content for Journaling
Per serving: 6 g carbohydrate, 0 g fiber

Actual Nutritional Content
Per serving: 125 calories, 6 g carbohydrate, 0 g fiber, 0 g protein, 0 g total
fat, 0 g sat. fat, 6 mg sodium

BLUEBERRY BELLINI

Instead of the usual (yawn . . .) peach Bellini, surprise your friends with a
delicious and fresh blueberry puree Bellini.

½ cup blueberries   2 cups Stellina di notte prosecco

Blend the blueberries in a food processor until pureed. Strain the pureed
berries to remove seeds. Distribute evenly into four Champagne flutes.
Pour prosecco into each glass.

SERVES 4

The Miracle Carb Diet Nutritional Content for Journaling
Per serving: 6 g carbohydrate, 0 g fiber

Actual Nutritional Content
Per serving: 135 calories, 6 g carbohydrate, 0 g fiber, 0 g protein, 0 g total fat,
0 g sat. fat, 1 mg sodium

APPENDIX A
STAGE ONE
GROCERY LIST

If your diet has been lacking in fiber, Stage One will gently introduce high-fiber foods to your digestive system. In time you will be enjoying fiber in its many varieties. Adding too much fiber too soon can cause discomfort, and that's not necessary. Instead, for the next two weeks you'll eat enough fiber to step up your metabolism while allowing your body to get accustomed to it. So dig in and stay focused. Stage One is intentionally simple, so there's no guesswork to trip you up. The great news is you won't be hungry because you are mandated to eat three full meals and one snack every day. Skipping them does not make the diet work faster; the idea is to eat every 3–4 hours to keep your blood sugar even and to prevent hunger. Going long periods without food will actually stall your weight loss because the body interprets lack of food as reason to store rather than burn calories.

HIGH-FIBER CRACKERS

HIGH-FIBER CEREAL (SEE APPENDIX B: MIRACLE CARB FOOD BIBLE FOR A FULL LIST OF CEREALS)

FRUITS (SEE APPENDIX B: MIRACLE CARB BIBLE FOR A FULL LIST OF FRUITS)

NON-STARCHY VEGETABLES (SEE APPENDIX B: MIRACLE CARB BIBLE FOR A FULL LIST OF NON-STARCHY VEGETABLES)

PB2

YOGURT, EGGS, AND COTTAGE CHEESE:

- 0% Greek yogurt, plain
- Fage Total 0% Yogurt
- Chobani Yogurt
- Stonyfield Farm Oikos Organic Greek Yogurt
- Light N' Lively Lowfat Cottage Cheese
- Friendship 1% Lowfat Cottage Cheese
- Axelrod Lowfat Cottage Cheese
- Eggland's Best Eggs
- Eggology 100% Egg Whites

CHEESE (WITH 0–3 GRAMS OF FAT PER OUNCE)

- Laughing Cow Light (all flavors)
- Kraft Natural Cheese, Fat Free Slices or Shredded
- Mini Babybel Light
- Athenos Reduced Fat Traditional Feta Cheese
- Friendship Farmer Cheese
- Part skim string cheese
- Fat-free or part skim ricotta
- Parmesan cheese (grated)

DELI MEATS (WITH 0–3 GRAMS OF FAT PER OUNCE)

- Sliced turkey breast (white meat)
- Sliced chicken breast (white meat)
- Sliced roast beef
- Sliced ham

FISH (FRESH OR FROZEN) (WITH 0–3 GRAMS OF FAT PER OUNCE)

- Salmon (fresh or canned)
- Tuna (fresh or canned in water or StarKist Flavor Fresh Pouch tuna in water)
- Catfish
- Cod
- Flounder
- Haddock
- Halibut
- Herring (uncreamed or smoked)
- Smoked salmon
- Sardines
- Sole
- Snapper
- Trout

SHELLFISH (FRESH OR FROZEN) (WITH 0–3 GRAMS OF FAT PER OUNCE)

- Clams
- Crab
- Lobster
- Scallops
- Shrimp
- Squid
- Oysters
- Mussels

PORK (WITH 0–3 GRAMS OF FAT PER OUNCE)

- Ham lean (canned, smoked, or boiled)
- Canadian bacon
- Tenderloin
- Center Loin Chop

POULTRY (WITH 0–3 GRAMS OF FAT PER OUNCE)

- Chicken or turkey (white meat, no skin)
- Ground chicken or turkey breast
- Turkey bacon
- Chicken or turkey lean sausage
- Cornish hen
- Applegate Farms Organic Turkey Hot Dogs

BEEF (WITH 0–3 GRAMS OF FAT PER OUNCE)

- Lean beef (< 90%)
- Round
- Sirloin
- Flank steak
- Tenderloin
- Roast (rib, chuck, rump)
- Steak (T-bone, porterhouse, cubed)
- Ground round

LAMB/VEAL/GAME (WITH 0–3 GRAMS OF FAT PER OUNCE)

- Lamb (roast, chop, leg)
- Veal (chop or leg)
- Duck or pheasant (Skinless)
- Venison
- Buffalo

DESSERT

- Sugar-Free Jell-O
- Tofutti Chocolate Fudge Treats
- Swiss Miss Sensible Sweets Diet Cocoa (25 calories)
- Attune Chocolate Probiotic Bar
- No-sugar-added Popsicle

COOKING SPRAYS

- Nonstick cooking spray

CONDIMENTS

- Balsamic vinegar
- Salsa
- Lemon or lime juice
- Wish-Bone Salad Spritzers or Ken's Lite Dressings
- Mustard
- Tomato sauce (Rao's or Healthy Choice)
- Nonnutritive sweetener
- Sugar-free jelly (Polaner Sugar Free with Fiber)

NUTS

- Pistachios
- Peanuts
- Almonds
- Walnuts
- Pecans

APPENDIX B
MIRACLE CARB BIBLE

STARCH LIST

Bread	Serving Size	Carbs (g)	Fiber (g)
High-fiber crackers	1 cracker	7	5
Bagel, 4 ounces	$1/4$ (1 ounce)	15	1
Biscuit, $2^1/_2$ inches across	1	15	1
Bread, pumpernickel, rye	1 slice	15	2
Bread, reduced calorie	2 slices	15	1
Bread, white	1 slice	15	1
Bread, whole wheat	1 slice	15	2–6
Corn bread, 2-inch cube	1 (2 ounces)	15	1
English muffin	$1/_2$	15	1
English muffin, whole wheat	$1/_2$	15	2
Hot dog bun or hamburger bun	$1/_2$	15	1
Naan, 8 x 2 inches	$1/_4$	15	1
Pancake, 4 inches across	1	15	0
Pancake, whole wheat	1	15	2
Pita, 6 inches across	$1/_2$	15	1
Pita, whole wheat, 6 inches across	$1/_2$	15	2
Raisin bread, unfrosted	1 slice	15	1
Roll, plain, small	1 (1 ounce)	15	1

Stuffing, bread (prepared)	1/3 cup	15	3
Taco shell	2	15	1
Tortilla, corn or flour, 6 inches across	1	15	1
Tortilla, flour, 10 inches across	1/3	15	1
Waffle, 4 inches square, reduced fat	1	15	1

Cereals and Grains	Serving Size	Carbs (g)	Fiber (g)
All Bran, Extra Fiber	1/2 cup	20	13
Barley, cooked	1/3 cup	15	2
Bran cereals	1/2 cup	15	5-14
Bulgur	1/2 cup	15	4
Cereals, cooked	1/2 cup	15	2
Cereals, unsweetened, ready-to-eat	3/4 cup	15	0-5
Cheerios	1 cup	20	3
Corn Flakes	1 cup	24	1
Cornmeal	3 tablespoons	15	1
Couscous	1/3 cup	15	1
Fiber One	1/2 cup	25	14
Flour (dry)	3 tablespoons	15	1
Granola, low fat	1/4 cup	15	1-3
Grape-Nuts	1/4 cup	15	2
Grits	1/2 cup	15	1
Kasha	1/2 cup	15	2
Millet	1/3 cup	15	2
Muesli	1/4 cup	15	2
Oats	1/2 cup	15	2
Pasta	1/2 cup	15	1
Polenta, cooked	1/3 cup	15	1
Puffed cereal	1 1/2 cups	15	1
Quinoa, cooked	1/3 cup	15	0.5-1
Rice, brown	1/3 cup	15	2
Rice, white	1/3 cup	15	1
Shredded Wheat	1/2 cup	15	3
Special K	1 cup	23	0
Sugar-frosted cereal	1/2 cup	15	0-3

(continued)

Cereals and Grains	Serving Size	Carbs (g)	Fiber (g)
Tabbouleh (tabouli), prepared	½ cup	15	5
Wheat germ	3 tablespoons	15	2
Wild rice, cooked	⅓ cup	15	1.5

Vegetables	Serving Size	Carbs (g)	Fiber (g)
Baked beans	⅓ cup	15	4
Cassava	⅓ cup	15	0.5
Corn	½ cup	15	2
Corn on cob, large	½ cob	15	2
French-fried potatoes (oven-baked)	1 cup	15	2
Hominy, canned	¾ cup	15	2
Mixed vegetables with corn, peas	1 cup	15	2
Parsnips	½ cup	15	3
Peas, green	½ cup	15	4
Plaintain	½ cup	15	0
Potato, baked with skin	¼ large (3 ounces)	15	4
Potato, boiled	½ cup	15	2
Potato, mashed	½ cup	15	2
Pumpkin, canned, no sugar added	1 cup	15	7
Squash, winter (acorn, butternut, pumpkin)	1 cup	15	4
Succcotash	½ cup	15	4
Yam (sweet potato), plain with skin	½ cup	15	4

Snacks	Serving Size	Carbs (g)	Fiber (g)
F-Factor Bar	1	27	12
Animal crackers	8	15	0
Chow mein noodles	½ cup	15	1
Crackers, round butter type	6	15	0
Graham cracker	3	15	0
Matzoh	¾ ounce	15	1
Oyster crackers	24	15	0
Popcorn (microwavable), no fat or low fat	3 cups	15	3
Pretzels	¾ oz	15	0
Pretzels, whole wheat	¾ ounce	15	2

Rice cakes, 4 inches across	2	15	0
Saltine-type crackers	6	15	0
Sandwich crackers, cheese or peanut butter filling	3	15	0
Snack chips (tortilla, potato), fat-free or baked	15–20	15	2
Whole wheat crackers, no fat added	2–5	15	2

Beans, Peas, and Lentils	Serving Size	Carbs (g)	Fiber (g)
Beans and peas (garbanzo, pinto, kidney, split)	1/2 cup	15	5–9
Edamame (soy beans)	1/2 cup	9	4
Hummus	1/3 cup	15	1
Lentils	1/2 cup	15	8
Lima beans	2/3 cup	15	5
Miso	3 tablespoons	15	5

Milk/Yogurt	Serving Size	Carbs (g)	Fiber (g)
Fat-free milk	1 cup	15	0
1% milk	1 cup	15	0
2% milk	1 cup	15	0
Buttermilk, low fat or fat-free	1 cup	15	0
Evaporated fat-free milk	1/2 cup	15	0
Fat-free dry milk	1/3 cup dry	15	0
Soy milk, low fat or fat-free	1 cup	15	0
Yogurt, fat-free, sweetened with no-calorie sweetner	2/3 cup (6 ounces)	15	0
Yogurt, plain, fat-free	2/3 cup	15	0
Yogurt, Dannon Light 'n Fit with Fiber	1/2 cup	13	3
Yogurt, plain, low fat	3/4 cup	15	0

Fruit	Serving Size	Carbs (g)	Fiber (g)
Apple, unpeeled, small	1 (4 ounces)	15	4
Apples, dried	4 rings	15	2
Applesauce, unsweeted	1/2 cup	15	1
Apricots, fresh	4 whole	15	1
Apricots, canned	1/2 cup	15	1
Apricots, dried	8 halves	15	4

(continued)

Fruit	Serving Size	Carbs (g)	Fiber (g)
Banana, small	1 (4 ounces)	15	1
Blackberries	³/₄ cup	15	5
Blueberries	³/₄ cup	15	5
Cantaloupe, small	1 cup cubes	15	2
Cherries, fresh	12	15	2
Cherries, sweet, canned	¹/₂ cup	15	1
Dates	3	15	2–3
Figs, dried	2	15	2
Fruit cocktail	¹/₂ cup	15	1
Grapefruit, large	¹/₂	15	1
Grapes	17	15	1
Honeydew melon	1 slice	15	1
Kiwi	1	15	3
Mandarin oranges, canned	³/₄ cup	15	1
Mango, small	¹/₂ cup	15	1
Nectarine, small	1	15	2
Orange, small	1 (6¹/₂ ounces)	15	3
Papaya	¹/₂ fruit	15	3
Peach, fresh	1	15	2
Peaches, canned	¹/₂ cup	15	1
Pear, large, fresh	¹/₂ (4 ounces)	15	4
Pears, canned	¹/₂ cup	15	1
Pineapple, fresh	³/₄ cup	15	1
Pineapple, canned	¹/₂ cup	15	1
Plums, small	2	15	2
Prunes, dried	2 medium	15	2
Raisins	2 tablespoons	15	1
Raspberries	1 cup	15	8
Strawberries	1¹/₄ cups	15	4
Tangerines, small	2	15	2
Watermelon	1¹/₄ cups	15	1

FRUIT JUICE, UNSWEETENED

Fruit	Serving Size	Carbs (g)	Fiber (g)
Apple juice/cider	¹/₂ cup	15	0
Cranberry juice cocktail	¹/₃ cup	15	0
Cranberry juice cocktail, reduced calorie	1 cup	15	0

Fruit juice blends, 100% juice	1/3 cup	15	0
Grape juice	1/3 cup	15	0
Grapefruit juice	1/2 cup	15	0
Orange juice	1/2 cup	15	0
Pineapple juice	1/2 cup	15	0
Prune juice	1/3 cup	15	3

Non-Starchy Vegetables *(One vegetable serving equals 1/2 cup cooked or 1 cup raw)*	**Carbs (g)**	**Fiber (g)**
Artichoke	0	6
Artichoke hearts	0	4
Asparagus	0	3
Bean (green, wax, Italian)	0	2
Bean sprouts	0	1
Beets	0	2
Broccoli	0	2
Brussels sprouts	0	2
Cabbage	0	2
Carrots	0	2
Cauliflower	0	2
Celery	0	1
Cucumber	0	1
Eggplant	0	2
Green onions or scallions	0	0
Greens (collard, kale, mustard, turnip)	0	2
Hearts of palm	0	2
Kohlrabi	0	2
Leeks	0	1
Mixed vegetables (without corn, peas)	0	1
Mushrooms	0	1
Okra	0	2
Onions	0	0
Peapods	0	2
Peppers	0	1
Salad greens	0	1

(continued)

	Carbs (g)	Fiber (g)
Spinach	0	2
Summer squash	0	4
Tomato	0	1
Tomato sauce	0	2
Tomato/vegetable juice	0	1
Turnips	0	2
Water chestnuts	0	0
Watercress	0	1
Zucchini	0	1

MEAT AND MEAT SUBSTITUTES

Lean Meat and Substitute (Journal as 0 grams of carbohydrate, 0 grams of fiber); 0–3 grams of fat, 45 calories	Serving Size	Carbs (g)	Fiber (g)
Poultry: Chicken (white meat, with skin), turkey (dark meat, no skin), duck or goose (no skin)	1 ounce	0	0
Cheese: 1–2% cottage cheese	1/4 cup	0	0
Grated Parmesan	2 tablespoons	0	0
Cheeses with 0–3 grams of fat or less per ounce	1 ounce	0	0
Greek yogurt: 0% plain	2/3 cup	0	0
Fish: Fresh or frozen cod, flounder, haddock, halibut, trout, lox, tuna (fresh or canned in water)	1 ounce	0	0
Herring (uncreamed or smoked)	1 ounce	0	0
Salmon (fresh or canned), catfish	1 ounce	0	0
Sardines (canned)	2 medium	0	0
Shellfish: Clams, crab, lobster, scallops, shrimp, oysters	1 ounce	0	0
Game: Duck or pheasant (no skin), venison, buffalo, ostrich	1 ounce	0	0
Processed sandwich meats with 0–3 grams of fat or less per ounce: deli thin turkey, ham, roast beef	1 ounce	0	0
Egg whites	2	0	0

Egg substitute	¼ cup	0	0
Hot dogs with 1 gram of fat or less per ounce	1 ounce	0	0
Sausage with 1 gram of fat or less per ounce	1 ounce	0	0
Beef (USDA Select or Choice grades of lean beef trimmed of fat): Sirloin, flank steak, tenderloin, roast (rib, chuck, rump), steak (T-bone, porterhouse, cubed), ground round	1 ounce	0	0
Pork (lean): Fresh ham; canned, cured boiled ham; Canadian bacon; tenderloin; center loin chop	1 ounce	0	0
Lamb: Roast, chop, leg	1 ounce	0	0
Veal: Lean chop, roast	1 ounce	0	0

Medium-Fat Meat and Substitute (Journal as 0 grams of carbohydrate, 0 grams of fiber); 4–7 grams of fat, 75 calories	Serving Size	Carbs (g)	Fiber (g)
Beef (most beef products fall into this category): Ground beef, meatloaf, corned beef, short ribs, prime grades of meat trimmed of fat (prime rib)	1 ounce	0	0
Pork: Top loin, chop, Boston butt, cutlet	1 ounce	0	0
Lamb: Rib roast, ground	1 ounce	0	0
Veal: Cutlet (ground or cubed, unbreaded)	1 ounce	0	0
Poultry: Chicken (dark meat, with skin), ground turkey or ground chicken, fried chicken	1 ounce	0	0
Fish: Any fried fish product	1 ounce	0	0
CHEESE (WITH 5 GRAMS OR LESS FAT PER OUNCE)			
Feta	1 ounce	0	0
Mozzarella	1 ounce	0	0
Ricotta	¼ cup	0	0
OTHER			
Egg (high in cholesterol, limit 3 per week)	1	0	0
Sausage with 5 grams of fat or less per ounce	1 ounce	0	0
Tempeh	¼ cup	0	0
Tofu	4 ounces	0	0

High-Fat Meat and Substitute *(Journal as 0 grams of carbohydrate, 0 grams of fiber); 8+ grams of fat, 100 calories*	Serving Size	Carbs (g)	Fiber (g)
Pork: Spareribs, ground pork, pork sausage	1 ounce	0	0
Cheese (all regular cheeses): American, Cheddar, Monterey Jack, Swiss	1 ounce	0	0
OTHER			
Processed sandwich meats with 8 grams of fat or less per ounce: bologna, pimento loaf, salami	1 ounce	0	0
Sausage: bratwurst, Italian, knockwurst, Polish	1 ounce	0	0
Hot dog (beef or pork)	1	0	0
Bacon	3 slices	0	0
Peanut butter (contains unsaturated fat)	1 tablespoons	0	0

FAT

Monounsaturated Fat *(Journal as 0 grams of carbohydrate, 0 grams of fiber)*	Serving Size	Carbs (g)	Fiber (g)
Avocado, medium	2 tablespoons	0	0
Oil: canola, olive, peanut	1 teaspoon	0	0
Nuts: almonds, cashews, mixed (50% peanuts)	6 nuts	0	1
Peanuts	10 nuts	0	1
Peanut butter, smooth or crunchy	½ tablespoon	0	1
Pecan	4 halves	0	1
Sesame seeds	1 tablespoon	0	0
Tahini	2 teaspoons	0	0

Polyunsaturated Fat	Serving Size	Carbs (g)	Fiber (g)
Margarine, stick, tub, or squeeze	1 teaspoon	0	0
Mayonnaise, regular	1 teaspoon	0	0
Mayonnaise, low fat	1 tablespoon	0	0
Nuts: walnuts, English	4 halves	0	0
Oil: corn, safflower, soybean	1 teaspoon	0	0

Salad dressing, regular, reduced fat	2 tablespoons	0	0
Seeds: pumpkin, sunflower	1 tablespoon	0	0

Saturated Fat	Serving Size	Carbs (g)	Fiber (g)
Bacon, cooked	1 slice	0	0
Butter, reduced-fat	1 tablespoon	0	0
Butter, stick	1 teaspoon	0	0
Butter, whipped	1 teaspoon	0	0
Coconut milk	1 tablespoon	0	0
Coconut, sweetened, shredded	2 tablespoons	0	0
Cream, half-and-half	2 tablespoons	0	0
CREAM CHEESE			
Regular	1 tablespoon	0	0
Reduced fat	1 1/2 tablespoons	0	0
Shortening or lard	1 teaspoon	0	0
SOUR CREAM			
Regular	2 tablespoons	0	0
Reduced fat	3 tablespoons	0	0

Beverages	Serving Size	Carbs (g)	Fiber (g)
Club soda or mineral water	8 ounces	0	0
Cranberry juice cocktail	8 ounces	36	0
Fruit drinks and sweet teas	8 ounces	25–35	0
Soft drinks	12 ounces	32–46	0
Diet soft drinks	12 ounces	0	0
Beer, regular	12 ounces	13	0
Light beer	12 ounces	5	0
Nonalcoholic beer	12 ounces	10–20	0
Daiquiri, margarita	7 ounces	33	0
Gin, rum, vodka, whiskey	1 ounce	0	0
Liqueur, coffee flavored	1.5 ounces	24	0
Tonic water/Collins mixer	8 ounces	22	0
Wine, red or white	4 ounces	2	0
Wine, dessert	2 ounces	7	0

Snacks and Desserts	Serving Size	Carbs (g)	Fiber (g)
CAKE			
Angel food cake, 9 inches, no frosting, from mix	1/12	29	0
Chocolate cake, from recipe		51	2
White cake, from recipe		42	1
Frosting	½ cup or recipe	26	0
CHIPS			
Potato	20 or 1 ounce	15	0
Tortilla	8–12 or 1 ounce	18	2
COOKIES, BARS, AND SNACK CAKES			
Brownie, from mix	2-inch square	25	0
Candy bar	1.75–2.0 ounces	30	2
High-fiber cracker	1 cracker	7	5
Cookie, from package	1 cookie	10	0
Graham crackers	1 sheet	11	0
Granola or cereal bar	1 ounce	20	1
Snack cake, cupcake	1 serving	30	0
FROZEN AND CHILLED SNACKS			
Fruit or juice bar	1 serving	6–23	0
Gelatin dessert	1 cup	38	0
Gelatin, sugar free	1 cup	0	0
Non-dairy frozen dessert	1 serving	20–50	0
Sherbet or sorbet	1 cup	50–60	0
Frozen burrito, beef and bean	5 ounces	40–50	5
Frozen pizza	7-inch single	25–50	2
PIE			
Apple, from recipe	⅙ of 9-inch pie	77	2
Lemon meringue, from recipe	⅙ of 9-inch pie	67	1
Pecan, from recipe	⅙ of 9-inch pie	85	4
Pumpkin, from recipe	⅙ of 9-inch pie	55	3
OTHER			
Caramel corn with peanuts	1 cup	35	2
Popcorn	5 cups popped	19	4
Popcorn cake or rice cake	1	7	0
Pork skins	1 ounce	0	0
Pretzels	1 ounce	22	0

	Serving Size	Carbs (g)	Fiber (g)
Pudding	½ cup	20–30	0
Pudding, sugar free	½ cup	12	0
Pumpkin seeds	¼ cup kernels	8	2
Sunflower seeds	¼ cup kernels	8	3
Trail mix	¼ cup	16–23	3

Fast Foods	Serving Size	Carbs (g)	Fiber (g)
CHICKEN			
Chicken pot pie	1	70	5
Fried chicken	1	11	0
Fried chicken, extra crispy or hot and spicy	1	20	0
Wings, any variety	1	12–14	0
Wings, honey barbecue, with sauce	6	36	1
Mashed potatoes with gravy	small	18	1
SMOOTHIE			
Smoothie, 24 ounces	1	90–140	2–5
AMERICAN			
Egg McMuffin	1	30	2
Filet-O-Fish Sandwich	1	39	2
French fries	medium	44	4
Fruit 'N Yogurt Parfait, 5.2 ounces	1	30	1
Grilled chicken salad with ranch	1	18	3
Hamburger or cheeseburger	1	36	2
Hotcakes with syrup	1	104	0
CHINESE			
Beef and broccoli	5.5 ounces	9	1
Egg roll	1	21	3
Orange chicken	5.5 ounces	50	2
Vegetable chow mein	8 ounces	48	4
PIZZA			
Most varieties	1 slice	29	2
Personal pan	1 pizza	71	6
COFFEE DRINKS			
Frappuccino	16 ounces	52	0
Caffe latte with skim milk	16 ounces	24	0
Caramel macchiato with skim milk	16 ounces	40	0

(continued)

Fast Foods	Serving Size	Carbs (g)	Fiber (g)
SUBMARINES			
Most sandwiches	6 inches	44–59	4
MEXICAN			
Taco	1 hard	13	3
Soft taco, chicken	1	21	1
Grilled stuffed burrito, steak	1	76	8
Nachos	1 order	33	2
Nachos BellGrande	1 order	79	12
Taco salad, with shell	1	80	15
Taco salad, without shell	1	42	13

APPENDIX C
ABOUT ENERGY AND
YOUR METABOLIC RATE

In order to lose weight, you must burn more calories than you take in. Your basal metabolic rate (BMR) is the amount of daily energy humans expend at rest. About 70 percent of the energy a human expends comes from the life-sustaining functioning of organs, such as the heart beating. Another 20 percent is burned through physical activity, and digestion of food—thermogenesis—accounts for the remaining 10 percent.

So how do you speed up this process in order to lose weight more efficiently? The secret to the Miracle Carb Diet is increasing thermogenesis, the Thermic Effect of Food (TEF), by eating high-fiber carbohydrates with lean proteins. These two nutrients take the longest to digest and actually burn calories during digestion.

FACTORS THAT INCREASE YOUR BMR:

1. Increased lean body mass
2. Regular or frequent meals
3. Exposure to cold temperatures
4. Fever
5. Caffeine
6. Stress
7. Pregnancy and breastfeeding

FACTORS THAT DECREASE BMR:

1. Loss of lean body mass
2. Skipping meals, dieting, or restricting food
3. Starvation or fasting
4. Exposure to warm temperatures
5. Aging
6. Lack of sleep

APPENDIX D
NUTRITION CRASH COURSE

THE FOOD GROUPS

Starches

Fruits/juices

Milk/yogurt

Non-starchy vegetables

Meat and meat substitutes

Fats

The great news is that F-Factor makes understanding the food groups easy and will change the way you look at foods forever.

I have divided the six food groups into two distinct categories: carbohydrates and non-carbohydrates. All carbohydrates contain 15 grams of carbs and average 60–80 calories per serving. Non-carbohydrates are counted as 0 grams of carbs per serving because they contain higher amounts of either fat or protein as compared to carbs.

CARBOHYDRATES (15 GRAMS PER SERVING)

1. Starch
2. Fruit/juice
3. Milk/yogurt

NON-CARBOHYDRATES (0 GRAMS PER SERVING)

1. Non-starchy vegetables
2. Meat and meat substitutes
3. Fats

Carbohydrates, Disaccharides, Monosaccharides: All carbohydrates contain sugar. The sugar in starch is called *maltose*, the sugar in fruit and juice is called *sucrose*, and the sugar in milk and yogurt is called *lactose*. Maltose, sucrose, and lactose are all disaccharides. During digestion, these sugars are further broken down into a single sugar molecule (monosaccharide) called *glucose*, which the body uses for energy.

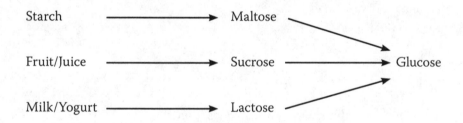

Glucose: Energy to fuel your involuntary and voluntary activities.

Glucose + Water = Glycogen

Glycogen: Your body's storage form of glucose. Glycogen gets stored in your muscles and liver.

Tanking Up on Glycogen: Think of your glycogen stores as dual tanks of fuel: one tank is your liver, the other is your muscles, and the fuel is the glycogen.

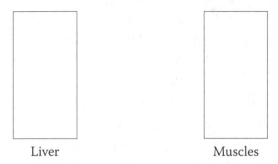

Liver   Muscles

Carbohydrates do not make you fat.
The excess of what your body can store as *glycogen* is
what makes you fat!

CARBS

1. **Starches:** Breads, cereals and grains; starchy vegetables; crackers and snacks; and beans, peas, and lentils
2. **Fruits/Juices**
3. **Milk/Yogurt (this does not include cheeses, cottage cheese, or Greek yogurt)**

Refer to the Miracle Carb Bible (see page 316) to see a complete list of carbohydrates.

NON-CARBOHYDRATES

1. **Non-Starchy Vegetables:** Broccoli, carrots, celery, leafy greens, etc.
2. **Meat and Meat Substitutes:** Animal proteins, PB2 (see What Is PB2? sidebar on page 60), cheeses, Greek yogurt, tofu, seitan, tempeh
3. **Fats:** Monounsaturated, polyunsaturated, saturated, olive oil, avocado, nuts

PROTEIN, NON-STARCHY VEGETABLES, AND FATS EXPLAINED

Protein (see page 322 for full list)
- **Lean Meats:** 0–3 grams of fat per ounce
- **Medium-Fat Meats:** 4–7 grams of fat per ounce
- **High-Fat Meats:** 8 grams of fat or more per ounce

Eating lean protein helps to preserve muscle mass during weight loss, keeping metabolism running at full speed. Your protein intake should account for at least 35 percent of your calories to increase satiety and facilitate weight loss. Some examples of lean protein sources are: egg whites, chicken, lean cuts of beef such as sirloin, fish, etc. See the Miracle Carb Bible.

Fish sources like salmon, mackerel, trout, tuna, and sardines boost metabolism. These sources of fish contain large amounts of omega-3 fatty acids (EPA and DHA, which are found in fish oil). Besides being incredibly healthy, omega-3 fatty acids affect metabolism and can improve skin health, reducing oiliness and helping to prevent breakouts. Omega-3 alters leptin levels (the hormone in the body that directly influences metabolism) and determines whether you burn calories or store them as fat. In other words, omega-3 increases the levels of fat-burning enzymes and decreases the levels of fat-storage enzymes. It's been shown to boost your metabolism by as much as 400 calories per day.

Non-Starchy Vegetables

Free food (as long as prepared without fat), i.e., tomatoes, cucumbers, spinach. See page 321 for a full list.

Fats

Monounsaturated: Shown to help lower your LDL levels (the bad cholesterol) and raise your HDL levels (the good cholesterol). Examples are olive oil, avocado, nuts, nut butters, etc.

Polyunsaturated: Some studies show that these fats may slightly lower your LDL levels. Examples are seeds, mayonnaise, margarine, vegetable oils, etc.

Saturated Fat: You want to avoid saturated fats in your diet as much as possible. Your diet should get less than 10 percent of its calories from fat, according to the 2010 Dietary Guidelines for Americans. This type of fat can lead to atherosclerosis and coronary heart disease.

AMERICA'S FIBER DEFICIENCY

Current recommendations suggest that children and adults consume at least 25–35 grams of dietary fiber per day from food, not supplements. The more calories you eat each day, the more fiber you need; teens and men may require upward of 30–35 grams per day or more. Yet the average American eats only 15 grams of dietary fiber a day. (To view a table of specific fiber recommendations based on age, gender, and estimated calorie needs, go to http://www.hsph.harvard.edu/nutritionsource/what-should -you-eat/fiber-table/index.html.)

For children, the recommended dietary fiber intake is 14 grams per 1,000 calories consumed. This can be achieved by eating more beans, vegetables, fruits, and whole grain breads and cereals. A gradual increase in fiber is recommended to minimize its side effects, such as intestinal gas. Remember also to increase your fluid intake as you increase your fiber intake.

FIBER AND ANTI-AGING PROPERTIES

Research has shown that eating high-glycemic foods—refined carbohydrates such as white breads and pastas—can cause a spike in blood sugar and lead to a process called glycation. Glycation, first discovered by the French chemist Louis-Camille Maillard in 1912, occurs when the sugar molecules in your blood become bonded to protein molecules, causing a chemical modification of the protein. Glycation reduces the flexibility and elasticity of collagen, which in turn leads to tougher, wrinkled skin.

To help you visualize how this works, bear in mind that glycation is also the process that causes pie and bread crusts to stiffen and brown.

APPENDIX E
MIRACLE CARB OPTIONS AT
POPULAR RESTAURANTS

P.F. CHANG'S

In China, meals typically consist of a healthy mix of grains and vegetables, with small portions of protein. When Americans adopted this cuisine, however, they made it far more meat-centric and whipped out their frying pans. Now "Chinese food" can easily become a calorie bomb with the likes of fried rice, deep-fried egg rolls, and crispy orange chicken. Nonetheless, it is possible to enjoy healthy Chinese cuisine at P.F. Chang's and avoid a bellyful of saturated fat. Just order any of these F-Factor approved items:

APPETIZERS

- Edamame
- Seared Ahi Tuna
- Chang's Vegetarian Lettuce Wraps

SIDES

- Spicy Green Beans
- Shanghai Cucumbers
- Garlic Snap Peas

SOUPS

- Egg Drop Soup
- Hot & Sour Soup

MAIN ENTRÉES

- Moo Goo Gai Pan
- Moo Shu Chicken (swap pancakes with lettuce cups)
- Ginger Chicken with Broccoli
- Beef with Broccoli
- Pepper Steak
- Chengdu Spiced Lamb
- Asian Grilled Norwegian Salmon
- Norwegian Salmon Steamed with Ginger
- Salt & Pepper Prawns
- Shrimp with Lobster Sauce
- Sichuan Shrimp Desserts
- Any dessert following the three-bite rule (P.F. Chang's Minis make it easy)

RUTH'S CHRIS STEAK HOUSE

Meat lovers rejoice—Ruth's Chris Steak House has got your number. This national restaurant chain is sure to satisfy your inner carnivore. But if you are trying to eat light, you'll want to watch your portions when ordering red meat. A typical New York strip steak here weighs in at a whopping 20 ounces—that's over a full pound of meat! Fortunately, at Ruth's Chris you can sit down to a lighter meal simply by ordering à la carte. Go ahead and order a 6-ounce portion of meat and a side order of non-starchy veggies—I promise you won't walk away hungry. Whether you are in Aruba, New York, Hong Kong, Madison, Wisconsin, or any other city with a Ruth's Chris Steak House, you'll find a great selection of menu items that are F-Factor approved:

APPETIZERS

- Shrimp Cocktail
- Seared Ahi Tuna (hold the sauce)
- Crabtini (swap the Creole remoulade for cocktail sauce)

SALADS

- Caesar Salad (dressing on the side)
- Steak House Salad (hold the croutons)
- Sliced Tomato and Onion (ask for bleu cheese on the side and just sprinkle a little for flavor)

SIDES

- Baby Spinach
- Broiled Tomatoes
- Fresh Asparagus (hold the hollandaise)
- Sautéed Mushrooms

MAIN ENTRÉES

- Lamb Chops
- Petite Filet
- Petite Filet and Shrimp
- Barbecued Shrimp
- Cold Water Lobster Tail
- Fresh Lobster

DESSERTS

- Any dessert following the three-bite rule

PALM RESTAURANT

Many people think of The Palm as a steak house, but originally this up-scale chain served only seafood. It's still a great place for seafood, which is naturally low in calories and rich in heart-healthy omega-3 fatty acids. There are plenty of fish in the sea, so you can afford to be choosy at The Palm. Pick from any of these F-Factor approved dish selections:

APPETIZERS

- Colossal Lump Crabmeat Cocktail
- Jumbo Shrimp Cocktail
- Sesame Seared Ahi Tuna
- Carpaccio of Beef Tenderloin

SALADS

- Mixed Green Salad
- Gigi Salad
- Monday Night Salad

SIDES

- Leaf Spinach
- Wild Mushrooms
- Asparagus Fritti
- Brussels Sprouts

MAIN ENTRÉES

- Double Cut Lamb Rib Chops
- Filet Mignon
- Broiled Jumbo Cold Water Nova Scotia Lobster (use lemon instead of butter)
- Atlantic Salmon Filet
- Swordfish Steak
- Veal Martini

DESSERTS

- Any dessert following the three-bite rule

NOBU

With locations on almost every continent, acclaimed Chef Nobu Matsuhisa takes Japanese cuisine to new heights of sophistication, with innovative specialties like miso-marinated Black Cod, Yellowtail Sashimi with Jalapeño, and Bigeye Tuna Tataki with Ponzu. At Nobu, any of the raw fish selections are bound to be extraordinarily good. You'll save a small boatload of calories, though, by ordering sashimi instead of a sushi roll, which is made with about a cup of starchy rice. When I'm at Nobu, I like to combine my favorite sashimi with any one of these F-Factor approved options:

APPETIZERS

- Miso Soup
- Yellowtail Sashimi with Jalapeño
- Bigeye Tuna Tataki with Ponzu
- Yellowtail or Salmon Tartar
- Shiitake Salad
- Kelp Salad
- Oshitashi

SIDES

- Kumamoto Oysters with Maui onion salad
- Bigeye & Bluefin Toro Tartar
- Ceviche
- Sashimi Salad
- Mushroom Salad
- Spinach Wrapped Sea Urchin

MAIN ENTRÉES

- Sushi and Sashimi
- Black Cod with Miso (ask for it to be served in the lettuce wraps)
- Filet of Salmon (light on the teriyaki sauce)
- Scallops with pepper sauce
- Chicken with pepper sauce
- Tenderloin of beef with pepper sauce
- Colorado lamb chops (light on the balsamic teriyaki sauce)

DESSERTS

- Any dessert following the three-bite rule

MESA GRILL

For American cookery with the flavors of the Southwest, look no further than Chef Bobby Flay's Mesa Grill, where dishes range from fiery and cool to sweet and tart. Bobby is a master at combining flavorful wet and dry rubs, robust sauces, and innovative cooking techniques to turn out exciting and polished dishes. Many of the barbecue items are bound to pack a lot of calories and fat, so your best bet is to go with simpler fare flavored with spice rather than sugars and fat. Enjoy delicious, healthy American fare with any of these F-Factor approved dishes:

APPETIZERS

- Sophie's Chopped Salad
- Sixteen Spice Chicken Skewers
- Barbecued Ribs (hold the peanut chipotle sauce)

MAIN ENTRÉES

- Mango and Spice Crusted Tuna Steak (hold the couscous)
- Wild Striped Bass
- Red and Black Pepper Crusted Filet Mignon
- Grilled Lamb Porterhouse Chops
- Cascabel Chile Crusted Rabbit

SIDES

- Smoked Chile Collard Greens
- Sautéed Spinach

DESSERTS

- Any dessert following the three-bite rule

PHILIPPE

Celebrity hotspot Philippe by Philippe Chow is famous for serving up superb Hong Kong–style cuisine, an exquisite type of cooking known for its lightness and layers of flavors, without any added MSG. Chef Philippe Chow is noted as one of the top Asian culinary masterminds of our time, with signature dishes like Chicken Satay in Peanut Sauce, Chicken Lettuce Wraps, Nine Season Spicy Prawns, and Peking Duck. Don't get caught up in the fried menu items, though. Instead, opt for any of these F-Factor approved dishes:

APPETIZERS

- Philippe's House Salad
- Spinach Salad
- Hot & Sour Soup

MAIN ENTRÉES

- Filet Mignon
- Chicken or Shrimp Lettuce Wraps
- Black Prawns
- Chicken & Broccoli
- American Black Sea Bass
- Live Maine Lobster
- Seasonal Vegetable Platter
- Philippe's Surf & Turf
- Steamed Whole Fish of the Day

SIDES

- Mixed Vegetables
- Broccoli
- String Beans
- Bok Choi

DESSERTS

- Any dessert following the three-bite rule

BICE

This famed Italian restaurant offers its guests the healthier side of genuine Italian food, made with fresh, natural ingredients. Italian cuisine has always relied on regional sources, and Bice keeps this tradition with farm-to-table practices, scouring local markets for produce, dairy, and herbs. If you are trying to eat light do as the Italians do, have an appetizer or side portion of any of their fresh, homemade wheat pastas, rather than have it as an entrée; you'll save about 750 calories. Follow with a lean protein that is either grilled, baked, or sautéed, then add a side of vegetables, and you have a perfect F-Factor meal. At Bice, F-Factor approved dishes include:

APPETIZERS

- Organic Mixed Green Salad
- Tuna Tartar
- Beef Carpaccio
- Chilled Maine Lobster
- Prosciutto with Melon
- Tricolore Salad
- Appetizer portion of the Spaghettini Primavera, Pelle All'Arrabiata, or Tagliolini Con Aragosta
- Minestrone Soup

MAIN ENTRÉES

- Pan Seared Filet Mignon (ask for a green vegetable instead of potato)
- Grilled Veal Chop (ask for a green vegetable instead of potato)
- Grilled Branzino
- Grilled Yellowfin Tuna
- Pan Seared Jumbo Scallops
- Grilled Organic Salmon

SIDES

- Sautéed Asparagus, Endive and Eadicchio
- Sautéed Broccoli Rabe

DESSERTS

- Mixed Seasonal Berries with Lemon Sorbet
- Seasonal Fresh Fruit Plate served with Mango Sorbet
- Any other dessert following the three-bite rule

STARBUCKS

With almost 1,300 locations throughout the United States, Starbucks is an American staple, offering a wide variety of low-calorie beverages and prepackaged foods. It's a great pit stop when you are on the go, but beware: A latte here can weigh you down with 300 calories, 10 grams of fat, and 40 grams of carbs. Calorically speaking, that's more than two cans of Coke! Best bet is to stick to basic coffee—a regular Venti coffee has only 5 calories and is fat- and sugar-free. You can always jazz it up with a splash of nonfat milk and sugar-free syrup. Or opt for any of these other F-Factor approved drinks and snacks:

MEAL OPTIONS

- Deluxe Fruit Blend Salad
- Starbucks Perfect Oatmeal
- Spinach Feta and Egg White Breakfast Wrap
- Chicken and Hummus Bistro Box
- Garden Veggies and Goat Cheese Bistro Box
- Chipotle Chicken Wrap
- Strawberry Blueberry Yogurt Parfait

BEVERAGES

- Café Misto
- Clover Brewed Coffee
- Coffee Traveler
- Pike Place Roast
- Café Americano
- Iced Caffe Americano
- Espresso
- Tazo Calm Brewed Tea
- Tazo China Green Tips Brewed Tea
- Tazo Green
- Tazo Orange Blossom Brewed tea
- Tazo Passion Brewed Tea
- Tazo Refresh Brewed Tea
- Tazo Shaken Iced Green Tea
- Tazo Vanilla Rooibos Brewed Tea
- Tazo Zen Brewed Tea
- Nonfat Cappuccino
- Skinny Caramel Macchiato
- Skinny Peppermint Mocha

DESSERTS

- Starbucks offers lots of Dessert Petites, which makes it easy to follow the three-bite rule.

DOS CAMINOS

Satisfy your Mexican craving without feeling like an overstuffed piñata. At high-end cantina Dos Caminos, restaurateur Steve Hanson has reinterpreted traditional Mexican fare with incredibly flavorful dishes such as ceviche, soups, salads, and fish. Lucky for you, many of the items on Dos Camino's menu are light and F-Factor approved:

APPETIZERS

- Traditional Yucatecan Chicken Soup
- Watermelon & Baby Arugula Salad
- Mexican Chopped Salad (hold the crispy tortilla)
- Jumbo Shrimp Cocktail
- Ceviche (any variety)

MAIN ENTRÉES

- Black Angus Skirt Steak
- Grilled Chicken Skewers
- Chile Marinated Red Snapper
- Jumbo Sea Scallops (hold the rice)

SIDES

- Sautéed Spinach

DESSERTS

- Any dessert following the three-bite rule

CHEESECAKE FACTORY

With locations in almost every state coast-to-coast, the Cheesecake Factory is perfect for a family night out. True, the menu reads like a novel—there are over 200 menu items to choose from—but thanks to their SkinnyLicious menu with items under 650 calories, it's a snap to eat great and still have room for some out-of-this-world cheesecake!

APPETIZERS

- Thai Lettuce Wraps
- Fire Roasted Fresh Artichoke
- Buffalo Wings
- Mushroom Lettuce Wraps
- Ahi Tartare
- Chicken Lettuce Wraps
- Ahi Carpaccio

SALADS

- Tossed Green Salad
- Santorini Farro Salad
- French County Salad
- Fresh Vegetable Salad
- Factory Chopped Salad
- Chinese Chicken Salad (hold the rice noodles)
- Herb Crusted Salmon Salad
- Seared Tuna Tataki Salad

MAIN ENTRÉES

- New Orleans Shrimp (hold the rice)
- Shrimp Scampi (hold the pasta)
- Salmon: Grilled, Miso, or Herb-Crusted (ask for green vegetable instead of potato)
- Wasabi Crusted Ahi Tuna (hold the rice)
- Grilled Pork Chops (ask for green vegetable instead of potato)
- Petite Filet (hold the French Fries)

SIDES

- Sautéed Snow Peas and Vegetables
- Fresh Asparagus

DESSERTS

- Any of their 50 legendary desserts and cheesecakes, but following the three-bite rule

Most Caloric Drinks	Calories	Carbs (g)	Fiber (g)
Margarita	740	56	0
Piña colada	644	90	0
Frozen daiquiri	400	45	0
Amaretto sour	300	30	0
Eggnog	300	30	0
Vodka cranberry	250	30	0
Gin/vodka tonic	200	14	0
Beer, regular	150–200	10–15	0

Least Caloric Drinks	Calories	Carbs (g)	Fiber (g)
Bloody Mary	120	5	1
Red or white wine	100	2	0
Distilled liquors (whiskey, gin, rum, vodka)	100	0	0
Gin/vodka and diet tonic	100	0	0
Rum and Diet Coke	100	0	0
Champagne	100	0	0
Low-carb beer	99	3	0
White wine spritzer	50	1	0

ACKNOWLEDGMENTS

There are many people whose dedication and hard work made this book possible. First, I wish to personally thank the team at Hyperion: Elisabeth Dyssegaard, editor in chief, for your enthusiasm and support of this book; and my editors, Gretchen Young and Laurie Chittenden, for your keen insights and skill at bringing my vision to the printed page. And special thanks to editorial assistant Allyson Rudolph for steering this project for us right from day one.

Thank you to my agent, the great Richard Abate, for your expert guidance and unwavering encouragement.

My heartfelt gratitude to my team at F-Factor: Rebecca Baer, Gerry Casanova, Kaitlin Eckel, Lou Mancuso, Tomm Miller, Jessica Rossman, and Shana Rubenstein. Each and every one of you worked endlessly and selflessly to help make this book a success. Thank you for your unwavering loyalty, commitment, and above all, your humor—it helped get us through many long days and nights.

Thank you, Gerry, for being my rock throughout the writing and editing process. Words cannot express my appreciation for your friendship and dedication.

Thank you, Rebecca, for working tirelessly on the manuscript, drawing on your extraordinary understanding of the F-Factor diet, as well as your clinical experience as a registered dietitian.

Jess, I can always count on you to be the first to offer to take on an assignment, stay late, and make things right. Your wit and heart will take you far in life. I am lucky to have you by my side.

Kaitlin, my little office general, thank you for coordinating the recipes, ensuring we always met our deadlines, and for keeping our place in order. I remain your biggest fan.

Lou, thank you for believing in F-Factor with your whole heart. You are a man of integrity. Thank you for all you do.

Thank you, Tomm, for your marketing brilliance and enthusiasm, and for being such a wonderful friend to me.

Thank you, Shana, for reading and rereading my chapters with the caring and critical eyes of a first-rate dietitian.

Thank you to my family for always being there for me. Thank you to my husband, Glenn, who has enabled me to follow my dreams, and to my three children—Tobey, Juliette, and Olivia—who make me incredibly proud and help me to keep it real.

Thank you to my girlfriends. Your love, laughter, and support are priceless.

And finally, thank you to my clients, past and present, who never fail to inspire and challenge me in the best possible ways. This book is for you.

INDEX

breakfast (*continued*)

    Creamy Mocha Smoothie, 219

    LEO Scramble, 220–21

    Mexican Omelet with Salsa, 222–23

    Sweet Ricotta with Crackers and Berries, 221–22

  Stage Three, 259–63

    Banana Berry Smoothie, 263

    Cinnamon Blueberry Muffin, 262–63

    Crunchy Cinnamon Swirl French Toast, 260

    Oatmeal Blueberry Pancakes, 259

    Spinach, Onion, and Cheese Wrap, 261

  Tanya's Toppers, 48

breast cancer, 24

broccoli:

  Blackened, 209–10

  Pesto Chicken, 279–80

  Soup, Creamy, 188

Brownies, Chocolate Chunk, 300

Brussels Sprouts, 212–13

burgers:

  F-Factor Cheeseburger, 284–85

  Wasabi Tuna, 290–91

butter, 81

Butternut Squash Soup, 272–73

cabbage:

  Asian Coleslaw with Shredded Chicken, 185–86

  Shredded, Soup, 191–92

  Vegetable Soup, 273–74

calcium, 81–82, 124

California Roll Salad, 183

calories, 12, 13, 15, 19, 20, 21, 26, 89, 90

  in alcoholic beverages, 144, 145, 147, 148–50

  exercise and, 87, 88

cancer, 5, 24

carbohydrates, 12, 19, 20–21, 26–27

  cravings for, 123

  high-fiber, determining, 80

  net, calculating, 27–28

  refined, 14–15, 19, 22, 85

  on Stage One, 30, 31

  on Stage Two, 54

  on Stage Three, 59, 60, 80

  on Stage Four, 85

cardio exercise, 7, 87–88

cardiovascular disease, 5, 14, 22–23

carrot:

  Cake Bites, 297–98

  Ginger Soup, 189

Cauliflower Soup, 166

cereals:

  approved, 62–64

  Hot, with Vanilla Drizzle, 182

cheese:

  "Bagel" and Lox, 180–81

  Cheesecake, 217

  Chicken and Red Onion Quesadillas, 276–77

  Easy Creamed Spinach, 296–97

  F-Factor Cheeseburger, 284–85

  Jalapeño Poppers, 251–52

  Mexican Omelet with Salsa, 222–23

  Raspberry Tartlet, 256–57

  Spinach, and Onion Breakfast Wrap, 261

  Sweet Ricotta with Crackers and Berries, 221–22

  Veal Parmigiana, 243–44

  Vegetable Risotto, 264–65

Cheeseburger, F-Factor, 284–85

Cheesecake, 217

chicken:

  Baked Apricot, 196–97

  Chimichurri, 278–79

  Cobb Salad, 225–26

  Coconut Soup, Thai, 192–93

  and Corn Chowder, 270–71

  Curry, 197–98

  Fingers, Crispy, with Tangy Mustard Dipping Sauce, 233–34

  Noodle Soup, 274–75

  Pesto, 279–80

  and Red Onion Quesadillas, 276–77

  Salad Spread, 175

  Satay, 234–35

  Shredded, Asian Coleslaw with, 185–86

  Soup, Grandma Claire's, 161–62

  Southern "Fried," 193–94

  Tequila Lime, 236–37

Chili, Turkey, 232–33

Chili-Garlic Flank Steak, 199–200

Chimichurri Chicken, 278–79

chocolate, 124

  Chunk Brownies, 300

  Cocoa Peanut Butter Flying Saucer, 213

  -Covered Banana, 299

  Creamy Mocha Smoothie, 219

  -Crunch-Coated Strawberries, 302

  Sweet Ricotta with Crackers and Berries, 221–22

cholesterol, 23, 90

Chunky Gazpacho, 165–66

cinnamon:

  Blueberry Muffin, 262–63

  Roasted Almonds, 254–55

  Swirl French Toast, Crunchy, 260

Cioppino, 289–90

clothes, 85

Cobb Salad, 225–26

Cocoa Peanut Butter Flying Saucer, 213

coconut:

  Chicken Soup, Thai, 192–93

  Macaroons, 258

cod:

  Cioppino, 289–90

  Fish Tacos, 286–87

  Steamed "Miso-Glazed," 203–4

coffee, 137

  Creamy Mocha Smoothie, 219

Coleslaw, Asian, with Shredded Chicken, 185–86

colon cancer, 24

constipation, 22, 24–25

cookies:

  Almond, 301

  Coconut Macaroons, 258

corn:

  and Chicken Chowder, 270–71

  Grilled Tex-Mex Salad, 268–69

  Mediterranean Couscous, 266

Couscous, Mediterranean, 266

Oven-"Fried" Artichoke Hearts,
210
Stuffed Mushrooms, 211–12
Zucchini "Carpaccio," 208–9
Stage Two, 250–54
Baked Zucchini Fries with
Marinara Sauce, 250–51
Balsamic Roasted Asparagus,
253–54
Jalapeño Poppers, 251–52
Not-So-Southern Green Beans,
252–53
Stage Three, 292–97
Easy Creamed Spinach, 296–97
Garlic Mashed Potatoes, 295–96
Hoisin-Glazed Eggplant, 293–94
Mediterranean Couscous, 266
Sweet Potato Fries, 292–93
Zucchini Pancake, 294–95
skin, 22
skipping meals, 49–50, 81, 112
sleep, 22, 56, 112
Slow-Simmered Marinara, 157–58
smoothies:
Banana, 219–20
Banana Berry, 263
Creamy Mocha, 219
snacks, 49–50
Cinnamon Roasted Almonds,
254–55
combining fiber and protein in, 49,
89
F-Factor Bars, 62
skipping, 112
on Stage Two, 57
on Stage Three, 67–70
Tanya's Toppers, 49
social situations and events, 85–86,
127–28, 135–36
alcoholic beverages and, 143–44
tips for, 146–47
see also alcoholic beverages
soups, 161–66
Cauliflower, 166
Chunky Gazpacho, 165–66
Creamy Tomato Basil, 164–65
Garden Vegetable, 163–64
Grandma Claire's Chicken,
161–62
Stage One, 188–93

Carrot Ginger, 189
Creamy Broccoli, 188
French Onion, 190–91
Shredded Cabbage, 191–92
Thai Chicken Coconut, 192–93
Stage Two, 228–33
Italian Minestrone, 231–32
Lentil, 230–31
Split Pea, 229–30
Turkey Chili, 232–33
White Bean and Escarole,
228–29
Stage Three, 269–75
Beef and Barley, 269–70
Butternut Squash Soup, 272–73
Chicken and Corn Chowder,
270–71
Chicken Noodle, 274–75
Vegetable, 273–74
Southern "Fried" Chicken, 193–94
Spicy Creole Shrimp, 207–8
spinach:
California Roll Salad, 183
Easy Creamed, 296–97
and Feta Egg White Omelet,
178–79
French Onion Dip, 176
and Ham Frittatas, Mini, 179–80
Italian Minestrone Soup, 231–32
Onion, and Cheese Breakfast
Wrap, 261
Stuffed Mushrooms, 211–12
Veggie Dip, 176–77
Split Pea Soup, 229–30
spreads:
Chicken Salad, 175
Egg White Salad, 174
Tuna Salad, 173
Squash, Butternut, Soup, 272–73
Stage One, 21, 30–52
benefits of, 31, 53
beverages on, 33
alcoholic, 50–51
carbohydrates on, 30, 31
dining out on, 51
fats on, 33
frequently asked questions, 50–52
journaling during, 31, 38–44
menu choices on, 44–47
protein on, 32

recipes, 178–218
beef/pork/lamb/veal, 198–203
breakfasts, 178–82
desserts, 213–18
fish/seafood, 203–8
poultry, 193–98
salads and starters, 183–87
sides, 208–13
soups, 188–93
shopping list for, 34–38
Tanya's Toppers, 48–49
things to remember, 49–50
vegetables on, 32
Stage Two, 21, 53–57
carbohydrates on, 54
exercise on, 57
frequently asked questions, 57
journaling during, 55
recipes, 219–58
beef/pork/lamb/veal, 238–44
breakfasts, 219–23
desserts, 254–58
fish/seafood, 244–50
poultry, 233–38
salads and starters, 223–28
sides, 250–54
soups, 228–33
snacks on, 57
Stage Three, 21, 58–82
approved foods on, 62–79
benefits of, 59
carbohydrates on, 59, 60, 80
desserts on, 73–79, 80–81
diet on, 60
frequently asked questions, 79
journaling during, 61, 79
recipes, 259–309
beef/pork/lamb/veal, 280–86
breakfasts, 259–63
cocktails, 303–9
desserts, 297–302
fish/seafood, 286–92
poultry, 275–80
salads and starters, 263–69
sides, 292–97
soups, 269–75
Stage Four, 21, 83–86
carbohydrates on, 85
frequently asked questions, 85–86
tips for, 84–85

steak:
   Chili-Garlic Flank, 199–200
   Fajitas, 285–86
Steamed "Miso-Glazed" Cod, 203–4
stews:
   Cioppino, 289–90
   Lamb and Eggplant, 281–82
   Texas Beef, 238–39
strawberry(ies):
   Chocolate-Crunch-Coated, 302
   Mixed Berry Daiquiri, 303
   Sorbet, Creamy Frozen, 255
stroke, 23
Stuffed Mushrooms, 211–12
sugar, 56
  cravings for, 123–24
Summer Sangria, 303–4
supplements, 50, 81–82
Sweet and Sour Meatballs, 275–76
Sweet Mango Salmon, 205–6
Sweet Potato Fries, 292–93
Sweet Ricotta with Crackers and
   Berries, 221–22

Tacos, Fish, 286–87
Tahini Dressing, 168–69
Tangy Mango Sorbet, 256
Tanya's Toppers, 48–49
Tequila Lime Chicken, 236–37
Texas Beef Stew, 238–39
Thai Chicken Coconut Soup,
   192–93
Thai Peanut Sauce, 160
thin person mind-set, 132–33
Tilapia, Blackened, 249–50
tomato(es):
   Basil Soup, Creamy, 164–65
   Chunky Gazpacho, 165–66
   Cioppino, 289–90
   Cobb Salad, 225–26
   Grilled Tex-Mex Salad, 268–69
   Italian Minestrone Soup, 231–32

Pork Pizzaiola, 240–41
Texas Beef Stew, 238–39
Turkey Chili, 232–33
Veal Parmigiana, 243–44
Vegetable Soup, 273–74
tomato sauce, 52
   Baked Zucchini Fries with
     Marinara, 250–51
   Hearty Bolognese, 158–59
   Quick, Mussels with, 204–5
   Quick and Easy, 156–57
   Quick and Easy, Seared Sea
     Scallops with, 291–92
   Slow-Simmered Marinara, 157–58
triggers and temptations, 126–42
   airports, 139–42
   attitude adjustment and, 130–31
   danger zones, 135
   movie theaters, 138–39
   outsmarting saboteurs, 133–35
   social events and, *see* social
     situations and events
   thin person mind-set and, 132–33
   tips for staying on track, 136
triglycerides, 23
Tropical Fruit Parfait, 181–82
tryptophan, 123
tuna:
   Burger, Wasabi, 290–91
   Salad, 173
   Sesame-Crusted Seared, 206–7
   Tartare over Mixed Greens, 184
turkey:
   Asian Lettuce Cups, 237–38
   and Black Bean Nachos, 277–78
   Breast, Herb Roasted, 195–96
   Chili, 232–33
   F-Factor Cheeseburger, 284–85
   Meatballs, 194–95
   Piccata, 235–36
   Sweet and Sour Meatballs, 275–76
Tzatziki Sauce, F-Factor, 283–84

vacations, 145–46
veal:
   Marsala, 202–3
   Parmigiana, 243–44
vegetable(s):
   Risotto, 264–65
   Soup, 273–74
   Soup, Garden, 163–64
   on Stage One, 32
   Veggie Dip, 176–77
visualization, 10
vitamins, 50

Wasabi Tuna Burger, 290–91
water, 33, 112
weddings, 85–86
Wheat Berry Salad, 267–68
White Bean and Escarole Soup,
   228–29
wine, 144, 145, 148–49

yogurt, 51
   Banana Berry Smoothie, 263
   Banana Smoothie, 219–20
   Creamy Mocha Smoothie, 219
   F-Factor Tzatziki Sauce,
     283–84
   Greek, Dips, 176–77
   Hot Cereal with Vanilla Drizzle,
     182
   Peach Crisp with Sweet Vanilla
     Sauce, 216–17
   Tropical Fruit Parfait, 181–82

zucchini:
   "Carpaccio," 208–9
   Fries, Baked, with Marinara Sauce,
     250–51
   Italian Minestrone Soup,
     231–32
   Mediterranean Couscous, 266
   Pancake, 294–95